WISE BEFORE
THEIR TIME

D0168114

WISE BEFORE THEIR TIME

People with AIDS and HIV
Talk About Their Lives

Ann Richardson
Dietmar Bolle

*With a Foreword
by Sir Ian McKellan*

Fount
An Imprint of HarperCollins*Publishers*

Fount Paperbacks is an Imprint of
HarperCollins*Religious*
Part of HarperCollins*Publishers*
77–85 Fulham Palace Road, London W6 8JB

First published in Great Britain
in 1992 by Fount Paperbacks

1 3 5 7 9 10 8 6 4 2

A catalogue record for this book is
available from the British Library

ISBN 0 00 627648 2

Printed and bound in Great Britain by
HarperCollinsManufacturing Glasgow

Contents

Contents

Foreword

Even after a decade of AIDS awareness, the world at large remains indifferent. Perhaps it's little wonder that ancient prejudices have been reinforced rather than weakened by a disease which combines the taboos of sex and blood, of sexuality and death. The mainstream media, until recently, have told too many lies. Governments, too, have been fatally reluctant to accept their responsibilities to educate and protect the unwary. Much of the time, it has been left to those who are directly affected by the virus, to organize and to help themselves.

At the fifth International Conference for People with HIV and AIDS, delegates recorded short autobiographies of their experience. This collection of their true stories is as powerful as any great classic of fiction. Everyone who reads *Wise Before Their Time* will come face to face with the greatest challenge of our age.

We are reminded that AIDS is a pandemic. Internationally, we await the antidote and the cure. Meanwhile, in the witness of these men and women from across the world, humanity is everywhere triumphant. Instead of self-pity, there is courage. Despair gives way to hope. Where there is anger, it is directed positively at ignorance and prejudice. The people who have written this book, far from accepting the status of victims or outcasts, modestly reveal themselves to be heroic. In their stories, the rest of us are challenged to re-examine our own lives as best we can.

Dominic, from India: 'I never knew what life was. Living is a treasure, it's beautiful; but you have to live in the right way – value everything around you. Not only people, everything, every moment. Life is fulfilling then.'

Ian McKellen.

Preface

This book is a testament to the belief of one man that people with HIV and AIDS, along with everyone else, can be the masters of their own destiny. Dietmar Bolle was diagnosed HIV-positive in the mid-1980s and died this January, aged 31. Following his diagnosis, he devoted his time to helping people with HIV and AIDS, both to control their own lives and to be recognized as having genuine expertise on their own condition. This book was his last tangible achievement.

There are now numerous books about AIDS. What is new about this one is that it is written from the perspective of people with HIV and AIDS *themselves*. It is they who know most deeply what it means to live day by day with a disease for which many are shunned and for which there is currently no known cure. They have been through the process of receiving the diagnosis, finding a way of telling their friends and relations, and searching for the strength to go on. This book is for those who want to hear what they have to say at first hand.

People with HIV and AIDS are often young men and women, who could feel highly vulnerable. Yet the central message of this book is the dignity with which they can face their situation. The individuals in these pages do not present themselves as 'AIDS victims' but talk instead of the joys of life and the fundamental values to which they have been drawn. It is this transcendence over their disease, not their vulnerability, which gives their voices real power. They have looked their own mortality in the eye and are *wise before their time* Whether or not we have any contact with people with HIV or AIDS, we can all learn from them.

But across the world, more and more people are coming to find that they know and, in many cases, love someone with AIDS. There are partners, parents, other relatives, friends, carers and sometimes children, all of whom may need help in understanding better what it means to be living with HIV or AIDS. Many feel completely alone, unable – because of the stigma involved – to tell others about such a connection. This book was produced with them very much in mind.

And it was also our hope that this book should bring strength to people living with HIV and AIDS themselves. Wherever they are and whatever their circumstances, they need to know that they are not on their own. Some have found this already – through the love of their partners, relatives and friends, through talking with others in support groups or through the kindness of those in the caring professions. But many remain silent and isolated – unwilling to admit openly the existence of their condition. Others are frightened to discover whether they have the virus at all, not yet able to cope with their fears of its consequences.

Some readers will already be knowledgeable about HIV and AIDS, for personal or professional reasons. But a very brief introduction may be useful for the uninitiated. HIV is the accepted shorthand for Human Immunodeficiency Virus, the virus which can lead to AIDS. A person with HIV may have few or no signs of illness. The presence of this virus can be readily identified and those who have it are said to be 'HIV-positive' or sometimes simply 'positive'. Once the virus has taken a certain course, which varies notably from one person to another, the person is said to have AIDS, shorthand for Acquired Immune Deficiency Syndrome. This is not a single disease, but a set of infections and cancers arising from a lack of immunity to illness to which the person with AIDS becomes highly vulnerable.

AIDS represents a genuine challenge for us all. The numbers involved are staggering. Each *day*, some 8–10,000 men, women and children worldwide become infected with HIV. It has been estimated that in 1991, some two hundred Europeans were infected each day and seventy new people diagnosed as living with AIDS. If current trends continue, there will be a cumulative total of forty million HIV-positive men, women and children in the world by the year 2000.[1] It is difficult to take such statistics in.

---

[1] These statistics are taken from a speech by the European Regional Co-ordinator of the World Health Organization's Global Programme on AIDS, September 1991.

It is the very size of the numbers that makes us easily lose sight of the *individuals* behind them. We need to recognize that those with this infection are just ordinary people trying to cope with their situation as best they can. And we may need to remember that they are to be found everywhere – out there, far away, and here, in our home town, on our street, perhaps even in our family. The individuals in this book speak for many, many others.

This book is both international in scope and personal in touch. We hear, among others, from Rebecca in England, Winston in Canada, Elizabeth in Uganda, Imrat in Malaysia, Roberto in Mexico, Erik in Sweden. They each speak tellingly about their lives – their fears, their joys and their coming to terms with themselves. Some are quite well off, some very poor; some have risen to the height of their profession, some struggle to remain in any kind of employment. Some live happily with a partner, some live alone. Most are fairly young, in their twenties or thirties, although a few are older. Their backgrounds are as diverse as that of any set of people grouped together solely by the coincidence of their medical history.

The idea for this book was first conceived in the course of planning the Fifth International Conference for People with HIV and AIDS. This took place in London, 11th–15th September 1991, with 550 participants from over fifty countries, all living with HIV or AIDS. It had the twin aims of enabling people to gain help themselves and to make others more aware of their needs. Dietmar Bolle was the principal inspirer and organizer of the conference. In that capacity, he had invited applicants to send in a 'personal story' for possible publication. I had been asked to write the conference report and, in the course of discussion, I proposed that we also carry out interviews with conference participants to complement and extend what they wrote.

This book is the result of these twin exercises. In total, roughly sixty people from twenty-two different countries submitted written stories of varying length. At the conference, we interviewed twenty-one participants from fifteen countries and all continents. We sought to include a good range of people, including men and women with differing backgrounds, ages and lifestyles. The one unavoidable bias in the stories reflects those attending the conference itself. Although open to anyone with HIV or AIDS, it inevitably attracted many people active in AIDS organizations in their respective countries. They tended to have found a way of living positively with their situation and to be seeking to help others to do the same. But we felt that to the extent that there proved to be a positive bias in these pages, so much the better, since this might serve as an inspiration to others.

The text in this book comes directly from the individuals involved. We have undertaken only minor editing in the interest of readability and confidentiality. With three exceptions, all names have been changed and some other details, such as places of residence or employment, have been amended to preserve anonymity. Of the others, two (David in England and Peter in the USA) expressed a strong wish for their real names to be used; the story of the third (Dominic in India) is so singular and had already been so widely publicized that it seemed inappropriate for it to be anonymized. A list of the people quoted, showing nationality, age and date of diagnosis, is provided at the end of the book.

A brief note on the shape of the book may be helpful. Chapter 1 is made up of four 'complete' stories, each describing a very different situation and together introducing many recurrent themes. Chapter 2 sets out how it feels to receive a positive diagnosis and some initial thoughts at that time. Chapter 3 describes the day-to-day process of learning to live with HIV, including efforts to remain healthy and continue with daily life. Chapter 4 explores the complex world of relationships with partners, parents, children and friends. Finally, Chapter 5 sets out some reflections on living with HIV and AIDS, including attitudes towards life and death, the role of spirituality and thoughts on the future. A poem, written by Dietmar Bolle during the last years of his life, sits as a postscript at the book's end.

I am very grateful to the Department of Health for funding the research for this book, and to Social and Community Planning Research for providing the research with an institutional home. Very special thanks go to Jill Keegan and Robin Legard from SCPR, who carried out the interviews at short notice with enormous sensitivity and skill. Christina Ball transcribed the tapes with great speed and care. Thanks also are due to Jane Ritchie at SCPR and Father Bill

Kirkpatrick for offering helpful comments on the final manuscript. But most of all, I am (and Dietmar was) grateful to all the participants who took the time to write about their experiences and to talk with great honesty to the interviewers about their lives. It is to them, and others with HIV and AIDS around the world, that this book is dedicated.

But I would like to end where I began – with Dietmar Bolle, my co-author whose own story is missing from this book. His obituary, below, tells of the public man, but a few words should be added on the private one. In his approach to his own personal life, Dietmar exemplified the very message that he sought to teach publicly – that there is no need to give up the search for both inner understanding and for life's immediate joys. He combined a dedication to his own personal development with a deep commitment to and capacity for intimate friendship. Even in his last weeks, he never stopped trying to learn, to challenge, to offer help to those closest to him – and to have fun. There was a will to *engage* with life which should serve as an inspiration to us all. It is what this book is essentially about.

Ann Richardson
April 1992

Dietmar Bolle

The following obituary was written by Tim Clark and published in the *Independent* newspaper:

Dietmar Bolle was diagnosed HIV-positive at Marburg, West Germany, in the mid-eighties, shortly before completing his training to be a nurse. At that time, Germany was debating mandatory registration of all people infected with the virus, even tattooing them.

Dietmar moved to the relative calm of London, but his response to this personal challenge shows the mark of the man who was to become one of this country's leading AIDS activists: he chose to nurse on an AIDS ward. The courage for such a brutal confrontation with one's own mortality is rare indeed, but he added the intelligence to turn that experience to remarkable and lasting effect.

As staff nurse at St Stephen's Hospital in London, he worked hard to improve the quality of care for people living with HIV and AIDS, creating model training programmes for visiting health workers. Through close friendship with a founder of Body Positive in London, his long involvement with that organization was strengthened. From the early days, he counselled newly diagnosed people, supported and advised volunteers, and shared his access to the latest medical news. He eventually became a trustee. This activism and the combination of his training, nursing experiences and his own HIV diagnosis broadened his understanding of how a strictly medico-scientific view of HIV/AIDS disempowers people. All his work thereafter reflects this conviction.

While still nursing, he took on even more commitments. He co-founded the Positively Healthy Trust to challenge conventional wisdom that diagnosis equals death. He advocated instead self-help, self-worth and self-determination, and the unbiased examination and evaluation of all conventional and alternative potential treatments and therapies. The early meetings were fuelled by his anger, principally directed at institutionalized fatalism over the course of the disease, and misdiagnosis and mistreatment of its many opportunistic infections.

He travelled back to West Germany to help establish its first National Body Positive Meetings there, an experience which inspired him to call the 'First International Meeting for People with HIV/AIDS' in London in May 1987. From that first gathering of fifty people with HIV/AIDS from ten countries grew today's global grassroots network whose last meeting, in September 1991, drew some 550 delegates from fifty-three different countries for five days of discussions on the growing abuse worldwide of the human rights of people living with the virus.

In November 1988, he also set up the West London Support Group – a network of mutual support for people living with HIV/AIDS, based in the area of the highest incidence of infection in the UK. But his great work, indeed his valedictory statement, and the celebration of all he had worked for, is the annual international conference following the first international meeting, which enshrines Dietmar's principle that those who are living with HIV/AIDS are those best equipped to determine their own present and future.

As those closest to him saw in the last months of his life, Dietmar Bolle had clearly decided to dedicate what strength he had left not to nurturing his own health, but to organizing and establishing these international conferences and their ongoing work all over the world. For this decision, although we may resent it, many of us have reason to be grateful. His achievements have changed people's lives for the better and, through the continuing work of these invaluable services, will continue to do so.

Dietmar Bolle, nurse and campaigner, born Ahlen, West Germany, 3rd November 1960, died London 11th January 1992.

PART ONE

Two Men,
One Woman
and a Baby

This is a book about individuals who live with HIV and AIDS. They are not statistics, they are not even a recognizable group. They are people with different personalities, circumstances and experiences. The best way to make them 'come alive' is to let them tell their own personal stories. What follows are the stories of two men and one woman, all living with HIV or AIDS, and a baby who died of AIDS a few years ago.

DANNY

Danny is thirty-two and from Northern Ireland. He is currently unemployed, having just spent four years at college studying theology. He had hoped to be ordained as an Anglican priest, but his ordination was deferred on grounds of his homosexuality. He is now seeking to have this decision overturned. He lives on his own.

Danny's diagnosis is very recent.

I was diagnosed HIV on 13th December 1990. The reason I went was I'd got a swollen gland under my armpit. I discovered that at Easter of last year and it was still there in December. When they took the test, it was a week's wait. Those seven days were like an eternity.

I remember it exactly, probably always will. The doctor said to me, 'As you know, Danny, we took some blood.' I said, 'Yes, I was here when you took it.' And he said, 'Well, we had the results back and I'm very sorry to tell you that it's highly probable that you are positive.' It was as if somebody kicked me in the balls. Then I thought, hang on, what do you mean 'highly probable'?

This was *my body* we were talking about. It took me three times saying I wanted to know what's going on before he said, 'Okay, Danny, the results of the first test are positive.' Although I'd more or less convinced myself that it was possible I was positive, it didn't really prepare me for hearing those words. I'd lived in hope that the result of the test would be negative.

I went with a friend, a close woman friend, for the results. I went out and got her and the poor woman, she knew right away what had been said. We sat and talked to the doctor. Or she talked and I just gazed into oblivion.

I went back to her place that night, to her and her partner. I intended to get totally drunk, but no matter how many drinks I downed, I couldn't quite make that stage. Who? Why? What's going to happen? Who can I tell? Why me? And even, 'Hang on a second, they got my test mixed up with somebody else. That's what it is, some other poor sod has been told he's negative and in fact he's positive.' And I thought, no, get a grip on yourself, that doesn't happen.

My health has been fine. I'm healthier now than I have been for the last two years. The chances are that I'd been living with HIV for at least two years, as my weight had dropped then, over three stone in four months. I did go for a test at that time – and that proved negative. They said to come back in three months, because I had put myself at risk, but I was so relieved I didn't bother going back.

One difficult aspect of learning about HIV is telling other people – friends, partners, parents and so forth.

The first people I told was the faculty at my college, because they were people I trusted. They'd seen me through the ordination being put off and stood by me. We disagreed very strongly, theologically, with God's view of sexuality, but that didn't matter. When I needed their support, they were there. They were fantastic. I couldn't have wished for more from anyone, both faculty and fellow students.

When I was first diagnosed, I was in a relationship with another bloke. We'd been together for a number of months. And although we practised safe sex, the first thought that came into my head was 'Have I put him at risk?' He wasn't around for a few weeks. When I eventually told him, all he did was get up and just hold me for about twenty minutes, which was fantastic.

We're no longer together. I don't think it was anything to do with the HIV, but it might have been. The important thing for me was his immediate reaction – wanting to support and comfort and hold me. He didn't get himself tested. He saw the health advisor and as a result decided that there was no call for him to be tested.

I haven't told my mother and brothers. The three of them know that I'm gay – they've known since I was nineteen. That caused enough problems in itself. I went home this Easter, not really sure whether I was going to tell or not. I was only there for a week. And when it came to the Wednesday and I hadn't told them, I thought no – thinking about my mother particularly – to dump this on her now and just leave would be an awful thing to do.

It's a difficult thing. What I don't want to happen is that in three years' time I become ill with something like pneumonia and end up in hospital. I don't want my mother to find out that way. That would be horrendous for her. But if I tell her now and then go on for the next ten years being healthy, will she spend those years in fear and trepidation?

In two or three years' time, I'll be ready. I'll know when it's time for me to tell. I want to tell her. It will send her up the wall, it will be as if things are caving in on her. After that, there would be, I hope, a tremendous amount of support.

There was a situation about three years ago where my brother wouldn't let me see his kids. That tore me apart. I'd arranged to meet him at his home, to be there for the evening. I met him in the middle of the road and he said his wife didn't want me near the kids, she's afraid of AIDS. He said, 'You're a queer, queers get AIDS, don't they?' I left him, went into town and just got totally wrecked. I was in tears.

One effect of telling people is that relationships can change.

Some of my close friends suddenly wanted to wrap me up in cotton wool. It was as if I became some china doll that had to be treated gently.

I was known at college as being one of the more controversial figures. I revelled in that. I'd be forever challenging people about issues to do with unemployment or race or sexuality. I loved getting into heated arguments at times. Two people in particular, I noticed that their whole tone towards me changed, they wanted to 'care for' me. I didn't need to be cared for in that way. I said, 'Listen, I'm still Danny, I'm not Danny-HIV-positive, I'm *Danny*.'

On one level, it was good to know their desire to shield me from other people's ignorance and fear. On another level, I'm a fighter, born into the civil rights movement in Ireland and brought up with protest almost running in my veins. It was the possibility that that part of me could have been lost. They became like the parent and I became the child. But I was able to say, 'Hang on a minute, I'm still *me*.' I still enjoy stirring things, I've spent my life breaking out of closets and I'm not about to be shut into another closet called HIV.

I'm now involved in a number of training groups. And I'll say, 'Listen, if I as a person with HIV get up your nose, then bloody well tell me.' If you begin treating someone as if they're breakable, then you're in danger of robbing them of some of their humanity.

There is always a fear of prejudice.

I get paranoid on occasion, I think I overhear or see the odd kind of look, as if people are talking about me, people whom I'm not close to particularly. I refuse to keep my HIV status under lock and key. I'm not broadcasting it from the rooftop, but one of the things about HIV and AIDS is the stigma and the loneliness and isolation.

I used to run a playschool. I really love kids. Often the mums would be a bit harassed and they'd say, 'Here Danny, take this little so-and-so off me hands.' And I'd take the child and look after them, while mum went for a walk. Which I loved. Sometimes, when the kids were coming through, before they'd get from A to B they would have to crawl all over Uncle Danny. You'd see me crawling under the tables chasing the kids.

One day, just after my diagnosis, I was doing that with one little kid and the thought hit me – how would his parents react if they knew I was HIV-positive? And I froze, it was a horrendous thought. Then I thought, no, I'm not going to let this child suffer. He's used to me chasing him around, he looks forward to it and I enjoy it as well. As for the parents, I don't know how they'd have reacted, because they didn't know.

A while later, I had an incident with a married couple whom I'm very close to. I told the husband I'd been diagnosed HIV-positive. The next day, his wife came with her child around the corner and she said, 'Look who's here, Jim' as she did every morning. And Jim came tearing round, 'Danny, Danny, hug', arms in the air. There was nothing out of the ordinary. Just this woman being the same with me as she'd always been. I walked away feeling twelve foot tall.

It is most helpful to meet others in the same situation.

I can come across as being very outgoing, easy, laid back. And I am, partly. But there have been times when it's almost as if the whole surroundings just freeze. And I'm just left there, feeling like I'm suspended on the end of some rope somewhere.

Within the week of being diagnosed, I went into the AIDS centre in my area and saw one of the workers. I told her and she didn't say a word, she got up and came over and held me. That was exactly what I needed. Then I found I was going in there almost every day of the week, just to sit down and have a coffee. And let people in the street walk past – they could be *out there*, I was *in here* and I was safe.

I asked if I could speak with someone else with HIV. The feeling of relief when I saw this person who had been living with it for at least five years and he was healthy! That was so good, to talk to him. We were in the same boat. He knew what it was like, he had experienced some of the same things and he was enjoying his life.

Just the other day, I was asked to speak to someone who had just been diagnosed. That gave me a great feeling of contributing, of helping somebody else, just like this person that I spoke to. Just being there.

Danny found he needed to come to terms with himself.

When I was first diagnosed, I felt very angry at myself, that I had been stupid enough to pick up HIV. I should have been practising safe sex for at least five years.

In one of my counselling sessions, the counsellor piled on top of one another five telephone books. She gave me a piece of wood and said, 'Anger doesn't have to be a negative thing, it can be healing, but only if you express it.' I started to hammer into the telephone books and it was frightening, the rage that was in me. It was directed against *me*.

My feeling about myself has changed. Overall, I like me. I am a wholer person today than I was this time last year. HIV brought out all kinds of issues – things that happened as a child – I've been able to look at them. I like being me. The God I believe in doesn't make mistakes.

The Jesus of the gospels and the Jesus of the Church so often seem two different people. Some parts of the Church even go as far as saying that AIDS is a plague sent by God. But those who think that haven't met my God. That's blasphemy, to say that God is a despot, playing germ warfare with sections of humanity, it's blasphemy.

I'm going to go ahead with the ordination. Very much so. I've been on the road to ordination for eight years and I'm not about to fold up.

DOMINIC

Dominic is thirty-two years old. He was born in Uganda, but his family moved to Goa when Asian people were expelled from that country. He lives with his mother and widowed aunt in a small village. At the time of his diagnosis, he was working for an environmental charity as a divisional organizer for Goa.

Dominic learned that he was HIV-positive after giving blood. What happened to him then was very dramatic.

My parents taught us to help society. Because there isn't sufficient blood in blood banks in India, for fifteen years I was a blood donor. The last time I donated, the blood turned out to be HIV-positive.

It was in December 1988. In February, somebody came to my house from the police and said, 'You're required at the police station, the inspector of police wants to ask you a few questions.' I was really taken aback. I was dressing to go to work. I said to myself, it must be one of my friends who is in trouble, who has given my address because I live close to the police station. I didn't have *me* in mind.

I went to the police station. They didn't know what to ask me, just 'Have you been sick recently?' I said, 'No, I haven't, why?' They said I had to go to the Panjan police station, the capital of Goa. So they put me in a police jeep and when I reached the police station, there was this police inspector. He asked me if I'd been abroad. I said yes. I was born in Africa and I had just come back from West Germany.

And then he said there were some health officials who wished to speak to me. They took me straight to the hospital, the casualty ward. There were doctors and nurses coming from various wards to look at me. I was really frightened. I kept asking the doctors,

'Why am I here? What is wrong? There's got to be some sort of a mistake.' The whole thing was bizarre. The attitude of these people was strange.

Then a doctor came in – I learnt later he'd been given some training on AIDS. He looked in my mouth, in my eyes and he asked if I was feeling well. I said, 'Everything's okay, why are you asking me these questions?' He never answered, but told the nurse to put my name in the foreigners register. Now, I am an Indian citizen and why should my name be in the foreigners register? This nurse brings the register and puts it on the table and there is this big sticker – AIDS. So that's how I came to know.

I knew what AIDS was, but I never really educated myself. I knew how it's transmitted, but I never practised safe sex. I had this feeling that it's not going to touch me.

I was so frightened, I felt no, this can't be. The other cases were all foreigners – isolated and then deported. I was the first Indian. The nurse said, 'Remember, you donated blood three months back? Well, the report returned positive and you have AIDS. They're going to take you to some place.' And I looked out and was terrified, because there were policemen with guns, big rifles, there. I couldn't see any prisoners or criminal looking persons and asked myself, 'Is this for *me*?'

I said to the doctor, 'Before you take me, please can we inform my mother, because she lives alone. She's an aged woman, she doesn't keep too well and whatever you are doing, you have to inform her.' They said, 'Don't worry, it's very close, we go and we tell her.' But they never took me there, they just put me in an ambulance with these policemen and took me to this former TB sanatorium. It was closed down, so they opened up the place and put me in there.

It was a nightmare – I was hoping to wake up. I was saying to myself, how are people going to react? And how long do I have – am I going to live very long? I'd had opportunities to read about AIDS and I never even bothered. So here I was lost, ill informed about the disease, and frightened because of the attitudes of people around me. My tummy was hurting me badly and I was cold everywhere. I was scared, very scared.

This was the beginning of a long period of detention.

The place was very bad, it had been closed for a year. I was the only person put in there. There was a layer of dust an inch thick everywhere. There were six beds, I had to choose the bed that had the least rat droppings, dust it myself and clean it up. They had to get someone to sweep and swab the place from the hospital. It was really bad.

My mother was able to see me only after twenty-four hours. She's a remarkable woman, a retired nurse. She came and sat next to me and said, 'They say you have AIDS. Don't worry, we'll see what we can do.' And that's where I broke down, started crying. I said, 'I'm sorry for the pain I'm causing you, I am sorry that it has to affect you.' And she said something like, 'We are in it together.'

They wouldn't allow anyone to see me unless my mother accompanied them, so it was difficult for me to meet friends. They were coming to see me and they just had to go away. I wasn't even aware that they had come.

I was angry with God – I am a Roman Catholic. I kept thinking – is this His way of making me pay for what I've done? I felt that it was promiscuity that led to me getting this virus. I felt this was God's punishment: 'Give me a second chance. Let this be a mistake and I will reform myself, I am prepared to make that sacrifice.' I was angry with everyone, including myself. There was no way to take the clock back. I knew that I could never lead the sort of life I was leading before.

The press were trying to see me. There was a big article about me, saying it has been alleged that he is a very promiscuous person, he has been seen on the beach many times with hippies and things like this. I was so angry – the hippy culture is almost dead in Goa and I don't know any of them. I said to myself, okay, everybody knows that I have AIDS, but I want them to have a clear picture.

I asked for a press conference in the sanatorium. I wrote letters to the newspaper saying, please send me your reporters, I'd like to talk to them. And when they came, I said, 'You're not making my case any easier. I am going through a very traumatic time. I'd like you to know how things stand. Educate people about it, because I want to go back home. I am not comfortable in this place, it's terrible.'

Things started improving from that time. There were articles, even in national papers, saying this person wants to go home. And about my mother, how she's so concerned, and the support from my village. Questions were asked about is it right that I am isolated. The Goan community in Canada – my uncle lives in Toronto – mobilized health clinics to send information to India. The Goan community in England also wrote to the government, saying that this isolation is wrong. Jonathan Mann [from the World Health Organization] sent some information, and the German AIDS Foundation.

From all this, I was quite well equipped with how HIV should be dealt with. So I called another press conference and said, 'This is how the WHO recommends that we deal with HIV. It has testified that isolation is no solution, it only drives HIV underground.'

A lot of positive things happened. People were writing letters to the papers, saying I should be released if my family, friends and villagers want. This was fantastic. But the government wasn't doing anything about it. The Secretary of Health said, 'Don't worry, he will be released very soon. We're just waiting for the assembly to meet and decide. Anyway, he seems happy over there.' That was their attitude!

After about forty days of isolation, I called my mother and told her, 'I can't take it any more. Let's go to court, let's sue the government.' We got a lawyer and he asked that I should be given interim relief and be sent home.

But this was not the end of Dominic's problems.

So after sixty-four days, I was given interim relief and allowed to go home. But I could not work, I could not leave the house. I was to be isolated at home.

I applied for one year's leave on loss of pay, because I anticipated this thing was going to take time. This was granted. We had a lot of postponements and after nine months, my court case came up. The legislation was changed from mandatory isolation [for people with HIV] to the option left to the health authorities. So, it was not a clear-cut policy. I am always afraid, they can isolate me any time.

In my court order, I am supposed to go to a health centre once a month. I was going to a centre, but it was a terrible risk exposing myself to other diseases. There was also the fear, if the doctor thinks there's something wrong with me, I will be isolated again. So I stopped going. But it is very dangerous, because I can be isolated for not reporting there.

The court order said that I could go back to work. I went back and was told by the chairman to get out. I couldn't understand his attitude, he was a doctor. I said, 'I'm going now, but I am not giving up my job. I have every intention of coming back to work.' In the meantime, they'd employed someone in my place on a permanent basis.

The chairman then got the three staff in the office to write to the head office in Bombay, saying they refused to work with me because I had contracted AIDS. One came to my house with the letter, saying none of them wanted to send it, but they were told that if they didn't, they would lose their jobs.

Then there was a new chairman. I told him that I'd like to return to work and he said, 'Come back any time.' I went back, but the former chairman continued to be a committee member and our office was in his hospital, so he had a trump card. He said he did not want the office in his hospital as long as I was there. New office space was found, but it was out of town and inconvenient. And I started finding that at committee meetings, the attitude was not very positive towards me.

I was asked to go see the secretary general in the head office in Bombay. He was very nice. He embraced me and said, 'Listen, we are getting a lot of letters, the Goa committee is not happy. We would like you to resign.' I said if the organization doesn't want me, I should not hang around. I felt terrible, but tried to be brave and smile. Six years I worked with this organization. I built my work up from scratch and this is what I get. Until I tested HIV-positive, everybody had a lot of regard for the work I was doing.

I used to draw quite a comfortable salary by Goan standards. But then I was on one year leave on loss of pay. The lawyer who fought my case didn't charge me anything, but I had to pay for his expenses – flights and hotels, it was a lot of money. I almost exhausted my savings. I didn't want to ask my mother – she would give me the money, but I didn't want to be a burden to her.

After I was at home for three months, I was approached by a couple to work for their bookstore. They pay me the equivalent of a little less than £20 a month. Even by Goan standards, it's very little. But I am grateful in the sense that the people are very nice, they all know that I am HIV-positive.

Dominic offers some reflections on his situation.

I have to live, I have to take it as it comes. It was very difficult in the beginning, but now I have learned to live with it. Being tested HIV-positive has made me very strong inside. I am able to cope with situations that normally people would not be able to cope with.

I go to this place in Goa, they have a retreat house right up on the hill which overlooks the Indian Ocean. It's run by the Jesuits and the director knows that I am HIV-positive. He said, 'Any time you are troubled, any time you have too much stress, leave whatever you're doing and come here and relax.' It's helped me a great deal. I now have a place where I can run to and someone I can talk to.

Before, I was a carefree person. I didn't value life, I didn't value friends, I didn't value simple things. I took my mother for granted, I took my brothers and my sister for granted. But now every contact with them is so meaningful. I believe that I have more depth. I am more loving, more caring and more concerned. I make people a priority in my life.

I never knew what life was. Living is a treasure, it's beautiful, but you have to live in the right way – value everything around you. Not only people, everything, every moment. Life is fulfilling then.

MONIKA

Monika is from Germany and is twenty-five years old. She lives on her own. She has known that she has HIV for six years, having acquired it, she assumes, from her boyfriend who was a former drug user.

Monika talks about her background.

I was a very protected child in an 'ideal' family. I was good at school. I had success in everything I did. On the outside, I had to be the luckiest child on earth. But I never felt that way; I was very unhappy. I felt that this was no life, everything was on track – straight, straight, straight.

Things outside that world were very attractive to me – being with somebody who had 'bad' experiences. My boyfriend was an ex-drug user. He was tested positive. In 1985, nobody knew how to handle the disease, there were contradictions in information. I was quite naïve and refused to think about it. I infected myself, half knowingly.

I made the test and it was positive. Then, there was a time of fighting in the family. It broke down their whole nice world. It was very hard for them. I wanted to show that I can handle it, that I'm strong. Because they had warned me, 'Don't get involved with a drug user.' It was a breakdown of everything. Not in the way that we didn't have contact, but we didn't talk about it, it was taboo. I had to pretend that I am just accepting it and that I can deal with it.

One year later, my boyfriend started to take drugs again, to shoot heroin. I can't now understand why – but I told him, 'If *you* take drugs, then *both* of us will.' And so I started to shoot heroin for about two years. HIV or AIDS was never a subject to us, it was just suppressed. When you have drugs, everything is okay, so why think about HIV? It didn't come close to me.

The whole situation changed when my boyfriend died suddenly. He didn't die of AIDS. He died on drugs, his body was just gone. It was a very big shock, because I really loved that man and now he was gone. I was standing there alone and all the problems fell on me.

I had to find my way out of drugs, out of denying my situation concerning HIV. This was four years after my test result. It took me about one year to fight my drug addiction. It was very hard time, very self-destructive – thinking and blaming and self-recrimination.

I started an apprenticeship and for two years I worked. Then suddenly, everything broke down. I just stopped, dropped out. I couldn't work. When my bosses learned that I was HIV-positive, they wanted that I go and I left. And the heroin wasn't there, so I felt that stress for the first time in all these years. I didn't receive any help from anybody.

Even the doctors I went to didn't know what HIV was. When I went to the hospital with a severe pain and told them I am HIV-positive, they didn't know how to react. They asked, 'What are you, pregnant?' They didn't know what this was until I said AIDS. I was one of the first examples of those strange animals in my home town.

From this point onward, Monika began to face the disease.

I moved to another city, because I was a bit paranoid about my anonymity. There, I contacted the AIDS Hilfe [AIDS Help – a support organization]. That was the first contact that I had with other infected people. I didn't have any self-confidence. I think it was a mixture of drug abuse and HIV depression. I really felt like there was nothing left.

And this was the beginning of the awakening. Was there a future? What about you? Everything had a question mark. The contact with other people in the AIDS Hilfe helped a lot. To appear normal, to see that I am not that strange animal, that extra-terrestrial. That I am a human being who lives in conditions that are a bit more frightening than for other people. So I came back a bit to normality and to myself.

I am working, I have a job three or four times a week with a small company. I recognized that I was always feeling walls, because they don't know my situation. They would understand me better, if they knew my background. So, I told my bosses and they reacted very, very well. It was an experiment for me and it changed everything. It's much better, I don't need to have that paranoia that they will find out one day.

I took part in a workshop with a lot of meditation for a period of a year. We were freer in that group. I tried to get inside, to learn to know the people. It did help a lot. Because you don't feel the victim of a virus when you see how much influence you can have over your state of mind, with your psychological processes. Like a self-fulfilling prophecy.

Sex and relationships.

Sex is another problem for me. My boyfriend and I never had to practise safe sex, because we were told it wouldn't matter – that a few thousand viruses more or less doesn't matter. So we never thought about safe sex.

Afterwards, it began to be a problem. I met many men with such a fear of being infected that it wasn't fun to have sex. It was just explaining, apologizing, 'I'm sorry, I'm HIV.' My sexual life just finished, stopped. I was so depressed that I did not have the desire to have sex.

And there's the question of guilt. When I look back, I have to keep myself from feeling guilty that I infected myself. Sex came to have a connotation of guilt. And responsibility. I think it's a typical woman's role – being responsible for somebody else. It is there when I have sex. What about the condom, if it bursts? There is always a little risk. The only responsibility was an end to sex.

That's very sad. Sex is, for me, a question of life and death. If I want to survive, I want to be there with my whole body. Otherwise it isn't life. I can't go into a monastery, that's what I *don't* want to do. I think it will change, but it will be hard work to get there.

There were also problems in friendships and with the family.

It took me about two or three years to talk to my best girlfriends about AIDS. I always had the feeling that I was bringing problems into other people's lives.

There are only very few people, two of them, who really got into it. The others see the facts and they tell nice sentences, 'Oh, what a pity, I wish I could find the words . . . . ' Often, they treat me as a child, 'Oh, poor Monika.' I don't want to be treated like that. There are only a few friends that are really caring about it.

You have a feeling that you are a living problem – just a problem on legs. You feel that you have to apologize: 'I'm sorry. You want to have fun, but there is a problem. You want to live and I talk about death.' That doesn't fit together with people of my age. They think about comedy, they don't think about dying.

My family are overprotecting. It's a problem for me. I know that this is a way for them to cope with it, because it's very hard for them. I just let them – if this gives them the feeling that they can do something, I accept it. But I refuse to be their little baby.

At the moment I am financially dependent on my parents. That is what I can't cope with. I want to be free, to be independent. That is a problem. But I don't have children and I can only imagine how parents feel about a child in this situation. And so I have to just let them.

Being around people with HIV or AIDS much of the time has an effect.

Sometimes I think I can't bear it any longer. It's too much, it's too hard. Too much dying, too much suffering, too much fear. That's always there when somebody's dying. That fear of your own death and suffering.

In the last two years, I hear so many people dying and suffering. A friend of mind died last week. It is a problem, not to break down. But all this confrontation with sickness and death has positive sides too. To free oneself from a certain fear of death. To see how beautiful it can be if somebody says, 'I am ready to go and I don't want to suffer any more.' It can be such a peaceful experience. It always hurts the absent, the goodbye.

You start to ask, 'What's after?' I think you need some religious thoughts or questions. I have to connect with something that's bigger. Some people call it God, some call it love or the energy potential. When you are faced with death, you ask these questions. You have to connect with something, just to get a little bit more strength or power.

I think there is a danger in the AIDS world. It sucks you in. You see just things going worse. People dying, make new friends, they are sick . . . . There are days when I just push wheelchairs through the city. And I say, 'Here you are, twenty-five. You want to live somehow, you want to enjoy something.'

After all these years, I have a great desire to enjoy myself. To just be light. And the situation doesn't allow me to. I know that there are people who derive much energy out of all this suffering. I don't feel that I am one of those. I am more depressed by it than activated.

Thinking about the past and the future.

I have changed a lot – in the things I am doing and how I think. There are things that I enjoy completely. Like sitting in the middle of London and watching red buses. It's my aim to be more aware of what's going on with me and around me. To be more in the moment, to forget about the future. Just to see time in another dimension.

I think my life has gained much more depth. I have changed from being closed to wanting to be open or be opening. But it's hard work. When you took drugs, you had long periods when you were really closed to everything on the outside. There are steps, I can learn.

I just changed my apartment. I am studying. I have to decide whether to continue my studying or look for work. I am very afraid about thinking about the future. I know that plans and positive actions can give you power, but I'm not at that stage. It is hard to make plans because one day . . . . It's something that holds you back.

Physically, my body works, everything's in order. I don't feel unhealthy. But I can't use my whole energy. Always there is a load of depression. I wish to change, I will work on it. There will be changes that I have to go through. Just having the opportunity to look at things I would never have looked at in a different life, I don't know . . . it's like a chance or a challenge.

DAISY

Daisy died of AIDS five years ago aged twenty-one months, having been diagnosed when she was just one year old. She lived with her parents and three older sisters and one brother. Her mother, Sarah, HIV-positive herself, had acquired the virus through Daisy's father from whom she is now separated. She had left an unhappy marriage some years before. None of the other children have the disease.

Her mother tells of the long wait to learn of Daisy's circumstances.

I knew from the first day I met my partner that he was bisexual, he was very open with me. But I hadn't thought about AIDS, because it wasn't really discussed. There wasn't much about it on television or in the newspapers. Most people who had it were gay men. I had no idea that I could possibly get it.

We were watching television about seven years ago – the man he'd been in contact with was telling everybody that he had AIDS. It was really strange watching this programme, seeing somebody you knew talking about this disease. We phoned immediately about a test and went to the special clinic nearby. The doctor wouldn't test me, because he said it was highly unlikely I would have the virus. I suppose he felt that women didn't get it having heterosexual sex.

It took six weeks until my partner was told he was positive. I rang up and the doctor just gave me the result on the phone, said, 'Well, yes, he's positive.' I felt terrified, absolutely devastated – and then I thought, well, I've got to be tested. And it was another six weeks – and we were told over the phone again.

Daisy was then eleven months old. Of course, we had to have her tested. That was awful, because we had to take her to the children's hospital. They couldn't get any blood – they were really trying and they were just hurting her.

And then six weeks later, I was told *she* was positive. We weren't prepared, they just took the test and that was it. We weren't offered any counselling, none at all. I was absolutely devastated. I didn't feel angry, I was just in total shock. I felt, well, that I'd done this to my child. Because I did. I believe she was born with AIDS, she had thrush when she was born. But because I fed her for a bit, I felt I'd given her the virus.

The sense of isolation was overwhelming.

It was awful because I couldn't talk to anybody. It was just the three of us, and I had to lie to my children. I just felt my life had come to an end. I didn't know how I could tell anybody about this dreadful illness.

My partner didn't want me to tell my parents about the disease. He wouldn't tell his either. He was very frightened. He was worried about how they would feel about him, they would blame him. I said I don't care, I need my mum, but he begged me not to. So for four years I didn't tell them.

It was dreadful. There were hospital appointments and I couldn't say .... They'd think I'd be having a nice day out and I'd come back shattered – especially when Daisy got ill. I couldn't even tell them what was wrong with her, why she was dying.

Daisy was fine when she was first diagnosed. She was really very well. Just learning to speak. She was a little bit late in walking. But when she was sixteen months old, she just stopped walking. I went to my GP and he referred me to a consultant, and they thought she might have a tumour on her spine. So they were testing for all these different things. I really believed that she had a tumour, I didn't think it could be AIDS.

We were in the hospital; I stayed with her for ten days. And one day this lady doctor came in and I said, 'Have you had any results back? Is it a tumour?' And she said, 'Well, you know what it is, don't you – she's got AIDS.' That's how we were told. I wanted to punch her. I've never felt so angry in all my life.

We were put in this room and the nurses were gowned and they brought Daisy's feeding bowl in and her spoon and they sterilized everything. I wanted to go make her a bottle and the nurse screeched at me, 'Get back in that room, you're not allowed out.' They were absolutely freaked out. They just couldn't cope with the fact that they had this child in hospital who had AIDS. They didn't know how to handle it.

And then they were bringing all these other doctors around. About ten doctors at a time from all over the hospital – nothing to do with paediatrics – just to view this baby. And that upset me.

One night I went home because I had to see to my children. The next morning, Daisy was just lying in a bed of blood. They'd done a bronchoscopy and burst the membranes. I said, 'What's going on?' and they said, 'Oh, we thought you could clean her up.' So they just left this little baby, eighteen months old then, in a bed of blood.

I was absolutely furious. I didn't care then. I just wanted to get out of that hospital. I said, 'I'm taking my baby home, I don't want anything more to do with this place.' I cleaned Daisy up and took her home.

The consultant was a really good man, but he didn't know anything about AIDS. We used to go see him once a month. He was very sympathetic and my own GP was wonderful, I couldn't have gone on without his support.

I didn't have much other support. Nobody else knew. Just my partner and myself. He couldn't cope with it. His way of coping was going to the pub, running away. But of course I couldn't, because I had this child who needed me.

I had ten months with no sleep, because Daisy became more paralysed and very twisted. The only way she was comfortable was on my shoulder. Some nights I would long for somebody to come and take this baby and just hold her for me. But you get an incredible strength. I could stay up all night, just walking with her and singing to her.

Daisy's death.

I told my parents Daisy was dying, but I couldn't tell them what was wrong. She became paralysed and I wanted to prepare them. I just said it's a disease of the central nervous system. Having to lie was awful. I really needed my mum at that stage. She'd always been there for me.

Gradually, Daisy stopped speaking. She became paralysed so that she couldn't sit up. She was in great pain, she had impetigo all over her, she had thrush, she'd get diarrhoea. She got pneumonia in the end. But the thing that kept me going was right up until three weeks before she died, the one thing that she could do was kiss. And at night when I'd be carrying her, she'd be going [kiss kiss] like that, as if to say, 'It's all right, Mummy.' That just kept me going. And her eyes. The last three weeks she was more or less comatose, but now and again you'd see something in her eyes.

My children were absolutely fantastic. My daughter would carry Daisy around on her shoulders, to give me a break. And my son was the only one who could get her to sleep, he'd sit rocking her little chair. And the two little ones, they did everything – they changed her nappies, they did everything.

I had told them that she was going to die. I said, 'Daisy's not going to live to be grown up.' And it was strange, because they were just so involved, they gave her so much love. They were amazing.

I knew in the morning. She was very cold when I got her up. It was a beautiful day, a really lovely sunny day. But I knew that was going to be the day. So I put on her prettiest clothes and got her comfortable. She used to lie on the settee on a pillow, so I could watch her. Her mouth was locked so I couldn't feed her, but I had a pipette and put it in like a little bird, just to moisten her mouth.

I put her prettiest clothes on and, well, I didn't leave her. And at six o'clock that evening I was cooking the dinner. My son was holding her hand and she'd gone very white. I said 'Get her father' – he was in the cellar – and when he came back he was holding her hand. And Daisy just died very peacefully with all of us there.

The lovely thing was that her body was so twisted – her feet were stiff and you couldn't straighten her legs out – and I just watched all that pain disappear. She became perfectly straight and she looked beautiful. Her blonde hair was like a halo, going round her face. It was lovely, because we had time.

I phoned my doctor and he came to certify she was dead. And then the children came and they all held her and talked to her. My little girl, she was only four, said, 'I think we must all say a prayer' and then, 'but I can't think what to say.' She made us laugh. But each in their own way said goodbye to her. I just said, 'Thank goodness you're not in pain, no more pain.'

My doctor had to inform the funeral directors that she'd died of an infectious disease. So when they came, they came in these suits and gloves. They just wrapped her in a plastic bag and took her away. And, well, it just was too much for me. I couldn't cope, I just had to run out of the room.

I'm not religious, really. I don't practise, but I've got deep-rooted feelings. And it did help in a way, because I was happy. I said, 'Daisy's one of God's little angels.' I missed her dreadfully because I'd had twenty-four hours a day of being with this baby. I loved the warmth of her on my shoulder, I loved carrying her around. It was like part of my body had been taken. It was gone and I couldn't replace that.

At the funeral, the priest got the children really involved. He wrote this lovely programme with very simple prayers and it just said 'goodbye' to Daisy. It was very moving. My little girl went up and sprinkled the coffin with holy water and they all laid their flowers. They absolutely adored Daisy. She was a lovely child – really sweet, lovely nature, very gentle.

PART TWO
Being Diagnosed

Probably everyone who has HIV or AIDS, as with any life-threatening disease, can remember the moment when he or she was first told about it. Some will have had earlier suspicions; for others, it comes as a complete surprise.

GETTING TESTED

Some people make a clear decision to be tested.

ERIK (SWEDEN)

In 1983, I started studying nursing and I decided I might just go and get it confirmed that I'm not HIV-positive. Earlier, we'd heard about AIDS, but not as a problem for us in Scandinavia. We heard alarm reports from New York and how it was a gay disease. Then the information got more specific, everybody could get it and you had to take some precautions. I just wanted to get it confirmed that I wasn't infected, because obviously I wasn't. I couldn't be. I had seen the pictures of ill people from America and I didn't look like that.

It was a shock, of course, when I heard that I was positive. But it didn't disturb my life very much. I talked to my doctor and he told me what I could and couldn't do. It didn't seem as if I had to change my life very much, just certain things when it came to sex.

My doctor was very concerned for me, wanted to give me all the help he could. He also was worried about my mental status, if I could cope. He said if I wanted to talk to someone, he would be glad to help me get in contact with someone who could give me professional help. He gave me a chance to explain how I felt. I was always welcome there. I was very lucky, I think.

MARK (CANADA)

I remember exactly where I was when I heard about AIDS the first time. I was in my parents' living room and a news report came on about how haemophilia and AIDS were linked. That was 1981 or '82. For about five years, it really wasn't a part of my life. I knew it was there. When I heard people talking about it I listened, because somewhere in the back of my head it seemed something I should pay attention to.

Of course, your curiosity builds and you hear more and more people are HIV-positive in your haemophiliac community. You go to clinics every six months and you sort of count the guys. So you decide one day that it's really past time. I really just wanted to get it over with. I had severe haemophilia and had been receiving blood my entire life, two or three times a week. It was 'Let's just find out that you are.' So many of us with severe haemophilia in Canada were HIV-positive, my common sense told me that I would be.

But when the doctor told me, that was the first time it had been told. It was like, you're finished, *fait accompli*. I couldn't deny it any more and it was going to be a real part of my life.

WINSTON (CANADA)

I was diagnosed in 1982. I was twenty-two years old. At that time in Canada, it wasn't a gay thing, it was the American disease. There was no name for it, men were dying mysteriously and they couldn't figure it out.

I was an IV [intravenous] drug user. I went because I wanted to know, I'm one of those guys that would rather know. I was going to be tested for a sexually transmitted disease, so at the same time I figured I'd have that test.

I got tested, waited two weeks for my results. I had no pre-test counselling. My doctor called me over the phone and said I was positive and I would live for three years.

I went to this community centre for counselling the following day. This guy was younger than me and he wasn't really concerned with what I was feeling – he was telling me about his last night's date. This went on for about fifteen minutes and I just got up and said this is not working.

I was really quite shocked and angry, how he did it. I also felt scared – like, is this going to be the end? Do I give up now? This is what he was telling me, *three years to live* – you've got a life-threatening disease, there's no medications for it. I was twenty-two years old, I was not ready to die yet.

Some people have the diagnosis thrust on them.

REBECCA (ENGLAND)

I think everybody who has had unprotected sex in the last ten years must deep down somewhere know that they are at risk from HIV. But there's a very big step from that to actually making a decision to have a test. I certainly never made a decision to have a test – I was actually diagnosed because I gave blood.

I gave blood in November and I knew that all blood would be screened for HIV. And I can remember saying, 'Well, I'm getting my HIV test out of the way at the same time.' I did marginally think that, but you have to fill out a very detailed questionnaire, so I felt quite happy about giving blood.

I simply got a letter in the post saying that I had tested positive on a disease that was transmitted by blood and would I come in to the transfusion service. I immediately thought it was HIV, because if it had been hepatitis or syphilis or something like that, they would have actually specified it.

(I'm pretty sure that I contracted the virus while selling blood plasma in Spain. The government had a system whereby they would pay people for their blood plasma and a lot of the people who donated were HIV-positive. The sterilization procedure was not good enough and some donors were infected by other donors who were positive. It was quite notorious, because some of the people who received the blood plasma became HIV-positive.)

I was totally devastated. My first reaction was that nothing would ever be the same again. I was absolutely terrified. I rang the transfusion service and went to see them on the same day. I had the diagnosis confirmed and got into a progressive state of panic as the day went on.

I actually registered a complaint about the way that I had been diagnosed. It was patently obvious that the doctor I saw at the transfusion service had never done it before – he was more frightened than I was. He wasn't able to answer my questions and what he did answer was not what I needed to hear at that point. I asked, 'What does this mean, am I going to die?' and he said, 'Well, most people do die.' Whereas I think the emphasis should be, 'We don't know what will happen, you might die or you might not, there are many people still living with HIV.' Just a little bit more sensitive to what you're experiencing.

MARY (ZIMBABWE)

I was first diagnosed in 1987. They did a test on me, because my baby fell ill. My husband was HIV-positive, they tested him before my baby. But he didn't tell me.

We took the child to the private doctor and then to the general hospital. He was suffering from bronchial pneumonia. My doctor asked for him to be tested for HIV and they did so – then me. The little one who is six months is not tested yet.

They did not explain to me, they just said that we want to diagnose you. They did not say which test. They just said they were going to do some tests. I wasn't knowing anything about AIDS or HIV before that.

My child was discharged after two weeks and my husband said to me that the doctor wanted to see us. We went to the general hospital and he explained to me that you are HIV-positive. I was so confused, I asked him, 'What does that mean?' He said that if you are HIV-positive, you have got the virus of AIDS.

Nobody helped me. They said, 'You are HIV-positive, but by 1995 you will die because it's a very dangerous virus which kills people.' I wrote it down, that in 1995 I will be dead. The doctor was in a hurry. All he said was that my husband mustn't give me another baby again.

PAVEL (CZECHOSLOVAKIA)

I was called by the hygienic service, the section on contagious diseases, to make a test. I can't understand why me. Maybe it was recommendation by police, because it was said that the police had a complete list of all gays.

I didn't realize very well what was going on, what kind of test, so I went without any warning. They didn't say what it was for, nobody said. They supposed that I knew about it, but they told me there's a blood test, something like that. And afterwards they called me to make another one, to confirm it. Well, it was suspicious for me a little bit.

I'd heard about AIDS, of course, but I had very small information about it. There was little information in my country at that time. It was written in the newspapers, it was very vulgar, a disease of gays, very much linked with sexual extravagancy. Gay people in the US especially. One of my friends made a trip to the US and brought back some newspapers. I read something about it, but I didn't feel concerned. I didn't see any connection.

At the hygienic service, they told me that it was positive. At first, I didn't realize . . . . It's only slowly you understand the whole complex of problems. There were two women – they were nice – they were not very used to saying it and one just showed sorrow. The other explained me that she was operated on for cancer and she's still living for six years. She showed me by her personal case that, well, bad things happen in life.

I was sent immediately to make the first test, immunology test. They told me to come regularly there. It wasn't very sophisticated in the psychological way. They didn't realize, for example, the need for confidential atmosphere. I was very afraid, because nurses were passing there and the wife of a friend of mine was working there.

They have now abolished the hygienic service. They were obsessed with one idea – to stop AIDS. Of course, we were considered the people who imported the thing from the West. It was very much ideological, because for many years in our country it was a disease of the West. It couldn't happen to us.

Some find out almost by accident.

ANGELA (SCOTLAND)

It was 1981. I had been up to Inverness to visit the grave of my daughter who had died a few months before. When I came home I was feeling really bad. My husband was already using drugs at this time. I was feeling really depressed and felt I had to get out of the house. He was sitting getting stoned with his pals and wouldn't go anywhere. I said, 'Do you fancy going for a drink?' and he said, 'No – have a snort and you won't feel anything. You won't be able to think at all.' And that's how it started.

Maybe two weeks later, I got curious about them using the drugs intravenously. I said I wouldn't mind trying it, just to see what it's like. I must admit he advised me against it, but I did it. From there, I did this every so often. At the end of nine months I realized I had a habit.

In 1984, I was seriously ill because of injecting drugs. I was in hospital for six weeks. I noticed they were taking a lot of blood tests, but I just didn't think anything. This is when I first started hearing about HIV. I left hospital thinking I was OK, but I remember having an awful lot of colds and feeling ill.

A few months later, I ended up back in hospital. I was in for a week and I think I must have got about ten blood tests a day. I wanted to leave the hospital – my mum had just died – and as I was leaving, the doctor said, 'You've got a virus in your blood

– we don't know what it is.' I didn't take it in as being the HIV virus. I used to say to people, 'I'm lucky, I escaped HIV and AIDS.'

In 1985, I asked my doctor for an AIDS test, because I was scared I might have become infected off my husband's injecting equipment, which he would leave lying around the house. My doctor said, 'Are you feeling ill?' and as I said, 'No', he told me to come back in January with my husband for a test.

In 1986, I was referred to the breast clinic. My doctor wanted to let me know what it would be like when I went there, if I needed the operation. He was going on about them being gowned up and masks and rubber gloves and I thought, 'What's he on about?' I just couldn't work it out and said, 'What do you mean, why is this?' And he said, 'Didn't you know you were HIV?'

BENJAMIN (UGANDA)

I started feeling sick and weak early in 1983, getting different symptoms – continuous fever, skin diseases, tuberculosis and general weakness. I moved from various private clinics to government hospitals while in a very bad state, but not knowing what it was I was suffering from. Even the results from my blood tests were not revealed.

In April 1987, I was admitted to hospital and told it was a TB problem. I had sixty injections for three months with anti-TB drugs. I was advised to continue with these for eighteen months.

I was attacked with typhoid in 1988 and re-admitted to the same hospital, undergoing a very hard treatment. I was discharged with a little relief for a few days, getting weak on and off. Later, typhoid re-attacked me and I was put on a drip for a week. I was just waiting for death. But this time I was lucky; the doctor had my positive results and advised me to join the Uganda AIDS organization.

I was shocked when I was told the truth that all along I had AIDS.

Occasionally there is a fight to get a test, particularly where a person is not viewed to be in an 'at risk' category.

KRISTINA (FINLAND)

I found it out last year, November. I had had an affair with a foreign man, from Africa. I read a newspaper article and there were different venereal diseases listed, with the symptoms. With HIV/AIDS, I started to search myself and I had that kind of symptoms. I just had an inner instinct that I could have it.

I felt that I should go to my doctor and take the test. I had heard of AIDS/HIV, but I didn't know about it. Well, I went to see my doctor and he said, 'Oh, no, Kristina, *you* don't need that test.' I started crying and I demanded that I wanted that test. I had that feeling that I might have it, I wanted to be sure – that I had it or I didn't have it.

Afterwards, I called the laboratory. I realized there was something wrong, because the lady there couldn't say straight to me that it's negative. The doctor said to me, on the telephone, 'There's something in that test, we sent it to our hospital, it's positive.'

No matter how familiar people are with HIV and AIDS, there may be little expectation of their own diagnosis.

DAVID (ENGLAND)

I was involved in AIDS from the beginning, almost the first person who died of AIDS here, I knew. I was very active in the gay community. We all began to look to how we could respond to this challenge which was affecting our friends. Which we thought was an American thing, would never really hit us here.

About six years ago, I went to South America. I used to go abroad a lot on my work. When I came back, I was very ill and I got put into hospital. Nobody spoke to me about what might be wrong, but there was a lot of whispering behind doors. And then the mother of one of the local children appeared at my door, and I said, 'What are you doing?' She said, 'Oh, I've just started work, I'm the HIV social worker.'

She sat down and talked. She told me that this was the ward for people with HIV and that someone had died there the week before. And then the doctor came in and talked to me about his work. He didn't talk about *me* at all. And all the time they were testing me for the virus. In the end, they sent me home. They said, 'Well, they've tracked down what it is; if it recurs, they'll have to treat it.' I didn't ask any questions. One didn't in those days, you didn't challenge doctors.

I had my only real bout of sickness in the US – I worked there for a year. I didn't have a test until I came back, about six months after. I was terribly depressed, my energy had gone and in the end I thought I must just know whether this was it.

I was stunned when I got a positive diagnosis, although why I should have been I don't know. The counsellor burst into tears – it was all friends by this time, I was at the heart of HIV work – as she said, 'I'm sorry, love, you're positive.'

ELIZABETH (UGANDA)

My husband, a civil servant, died in November 1989, coming to fifty-two years. I suspect he must have died of AIDS, but during the time of his sickness, I was busy, I didn't have time to find out.

It started in 1980, he came out with wounds in his head. When he went to hospital, they said it was a sort of psoriasis, so we took it as just a skin disease. He tried a number of medicines, but nothing could help. At first, he was healthy apart from that problem. As time went on, he started experiencing skin rash over the body. One doctor, in 1985, told him that such skin problems couldn't be cured.

But he kept on, he kept on trying. He used to go to Europe on work and got some better medicines there. They could temporarily help, but still couldn't heal him completely. He also tried local herbs. In 1989, he went down with malaria, which really weakened him. And then the doctors were treating one disease after another until the entire body became so weak that he was bedridden.

On 8th November, he passed away. I will never know if he suspected AIDS. He must have known that it was that disease, but didn't know how to tell me because of the way I would have reacted. But I had already forgiven him for whatever had gone on. If he knew that his mischief would lead to death, he wouldn't have kept the way he did. God demands us to forgive each other. I forgave him and nursed him up to the very last.

After his death, it was nine months before I went for a test. I thought it was obvious that I had it – if he had it, automatically I must be having it. We were together all the time and we loved each other, so obviously I knew I had it. And I had no time.

I used to hear stories that in some cases, husbands have died and their women have been proved negative. Deep in the bottom of my heart, I knew it was impossible, but I just wanted to prove what people say. That's why I went, with the hope that maybe I could be one of those lucky ones.

I was already a born-again Christian. We believe in divine healing, so I knew I was in the hands of Jesus, the son of God our creator. I believed that now I was in the Lord's hands and if I went on praying, He would heal me, so I was not offended by the positive results.

Sometimes the situation is not fully understood.

ANGELINA (UGANDA)

It was after the ninth month that I realized all was not well with my child. She had just completed her inoculations, but she was always sickly. I went from one hospital to another to no avail, until one doctor got concerned and had our blood taken without explaining why. When I next contacted him, his attitude towards us had changed. As he looked up our records, he commented to his colleague, 'Why bother if they are positive? Don't waste your time.'

This was at a busy out-patients clinic where doctors share rooms. It puzzled me, but I dared not venture further. He made up a prescription and sent us off. I decided not to see him again.

I had to take on extra responsibility, an influx of displaced relatives had joined me. I became so preoccupied that I overlooked my child's health. It was during the induction course for a new counselling job, while being given the facts about HIV/AIDS, that my suspicions were aroused about my child's possible infection.

I revealed my fears to the counselling trainer, a kind and understanding lady who personally came home to appraise the child. With her help and support I was able to face the inevitable. My blood and the baby's was taken again. My worst fears were proved right when our results turned out positive. The kind paediatrician offered us help and support even after she knew our status.

And here is one semi-humorous account of a long diagnosis:

DEREK (ENGLAND)

It started in early January this year. I developed what I thought was the beginnings of an abscess, so off to the dentist I go. 'Yes, it looks like an abscess.' After three weeks or so of different treatments, the dentist referred me to the dental hospital: 'Yes, it's an abscess, don't understand its lack of response to treatment.' After a painful exploration, I was sent away on another course of antibiotics. 'Come back in two weeks.'

Still no success, and by now my 'abscess' had doubled in size. 'Very interesting, can't think what it is. Do you mind if my colleagues have a look?' – a phrase that was later to become a nightmare – 'We'll do a biopsy.' Which they did. 'Come back in two weeks.'

Two weeks passed and the thing had doubled in size and my teeth were becoming loose. 'We haven't actually got final results, but preliminary investigation rules out anything malignant, which I'm sure you were worried about. Do you mind if I fetch a colleague to take a look? Can you come back in two weeks?'

The thing doubled in size again and expanded to the palate. It also lifted away from the teeth exposing roots and causing toothache. I could no longer eat properly and became good friends with the paracetamol bottle. 'Hello, how are things? Oh dear, it has got bigger. Well, the good news is the full biopsy report says it's definitely not malignant. The bad news is we still don't know what it is. If it proves a problem, we'll have you in and operate. Do you mind if I bring some colleagues to have a look at it? [*Bring the whole flipping hospital – somebody must know what it is.*] Can you come back in a month?'

A week or so passes. I can't eat or sleep. My bills for paracetamol will be bigger than the NHS budget. My social life has gone to pot and I'm snapping at everyone at work. 'Can I come in? This thing is driving me crazy.' Chat to nurse while waiting. 'Well, you're in the hands of experts here. They know what they're doing.' [*If the experts don't know, what else am I supposed to do?*] 'Hello, there, I believe you're having some problems. Oh, it does appear to have grown. Can I fetch some colleagues? [*Why not? Let's have a party!*] We need to do something quickly. [*At last!*] We'll have you in and operate. Can you come back next week?'

'Hello, there. Well, it seems to be malignant after all, but on a scale of 0–10, it's probably about 5. [*So, what are you telling me?*] Can I bring in a colleague? [*Please do.*] I don't like to use the word "cancer" these days, people imagine all sorts of things. [*Too flipping right, call it what you want, but give me some facts.*] Can I bring in another colleague?' [*Please do, what's he going to call it?*]

'Are you sitting comfortably? We have to ask you this question, so don't be offended. [*Damn.*] Are you or have you ever been homosexual or bisexual?' [*Double damn! I should have seen this coming.*] 'Well, yes, I was, I still am.' 'This sort of thing has been seen in these groups of people. We'd like you to speak to

Professor E.' [*Are you trying to tell me what I think?*] They are. 'We'd like you to take an HIV test. [*Triple damn.*] Don't worry, it's all confidential.'

'Hello, there. Yes, it's Karposi's Sarcoma. You've got AIDS. Can I bring in some of my colleagues?'

TELLING OTHER PEOPLE

One of the first questions on being diagnosed is who to tell. There can be very reassuring reactions.

IMRAT (MALAYSIA)

I went to Australia and, for the first three months there, I was losing weight and had diarrhoea and terrible flu. Two months after, I was still losing weight. The doctor put us to another doctor, who said that we'll probably have to run an AIDS test.

In Malaysia at that time, AIDS did not exist, nobody talked about it. Of course, we heard about it in the papers, it's an epidemic hitting the US, but we had not had any cases or nobody knew about them. So the first thing I told the doctor, 'Look,' I said, 'as far as I'm concerned we Malaysians don't get AIDS.'

I went for the test, and one week after the results came back positive. The only knowledge I had at that time was if you have AIDS you die – you have no hopes. I was confused, depressed, really terrified. I said that's it, I probably have a month or two months to live.

I called my family. I told them I'm sick, I'm not feeling well and I probably have this thing called AIDS. The immediate reaction was – I'm the only son in the family – my brother-in-law flew down from Singapore. He didn't talk to me about being gay or having AIDS, he just ignored the whole topic. The main concern was to bring me back home.

He booked a flight the next day. It was quite depressing. I was crying all the way, trying to think how will I face my family. Because I knew that my whole family will be there, waiting for me to come back. I was not ashamed of what I had, it was more talking to them about it. They'd probably think that I did something sinful, something that's dirty. This is what I was afraid of, facing them.

I was really surprised when we came in the airport. My mum was there, my dad, my sisters, they all came and hugged me and they saw how weak I was. I think they had the same idea as I had – that I'm going to die.

PETER (USA)

It was difficult to tell my lover I had HIV. I did it on the very first trip that he came to visit, about six weeks after I'd found out. I had presumed that as soon as he knew, he would walk out. His reaction, after we had discussed it, was where would I walk *to*? It was very endearing, made us much closer, there's no question about that.

When I decided that I would tell, everybody was going to be told. I made no list. Because I knew that if I tell one person, that person may just run into another person and so on. If they are truly friends, they're entitled to my well-being and they're also entitled to my bad-being or my worst-being.

The one unfortunate part was that before I could tell my mother and sister, a friend of mine – former friend – decided to tell them instead. I had not counted on that happening. If I'm going to tell somebody that I'm HIV-positive, I want to tell them in person. When I see the reaction, I can cater to it. My sister phoned and said, 'Is this true?' and I said, 'Well, I'm afraid that it is and I'm very sorry and very angry because I wanted to tell you in person. Please forgive me.' And the result is that my mother and sister and I are much closer than we were ever before. And we were already very close.

ERIK (SWEDEN)

On the second day, I talked to my best friend about it. She was a woman, twenty years older than me, with two sons nearly my age. We met in nursing school and we had a really good friendship. I often stayed with them, because we studied together. I actually went into their family in a way.

I talked to her about it and she was sad at first. And then she said, 'Well, we just have to take some precautions, that's all – if you forget your shaving things at home, you don't borrow the boys' and so on.' And, just practical things, if I cut myself in the kitchen, she said just find out what we should do. She was a great help to me.

But there can also be very negative reactions.

ANGELA (SCOTLAND)

After I left the doctors, I went home to tell my husband. I went into the house, he was sitting at the fire. I said, 'I've got something to tell you, I've been told that I've got HIV.' He said, 'And how do they know? How did they find out? So you've got HIV and the doctors are just telling you now! And I've been sleeping with you all this time. I've been in gaol, so it's impossible that I've given it to you. You must have given it to me.' Well, he is non-tested so he doesn't even know.

There was no concern on his part really, he was just so angry. He put all the blame on me. He went on and on and said, 'You'd better get the doctors sued.' That was his concern, get the doctors sued. And then, 'You'd better not let anybody know.' He didn't want people to know that there was a chance that he had it, so I was to keep my mouth shut about myself. I wasn't to tell anybody and that was it.

I just felt really hurt. This man is supposed to love me and I don't know how he can love anybody, treating me like that, making me feel like a leper. He's supposed to be the closest person to me and he doesn't want that I tell anybody else. It was just so scary.

Sometimes the reaction, although meant kindly, is hard to take.

DAVID (ENGLAND)

My ex-lover came rushing back – someone had told him that I'd got this diagnosis – and he wanted me to go to bed and be a 'victim'. He was going to look after me and we were just going to have two or three friends, you mustn't tell your mother, all this stuff.

I was just letting it all happen – and yet I was running a training programme for people with HIV. So I was getting challenged by my philosophy in my own personal life. That first month or two, I was not living that challenge. I was allowing this person to take over and disempower me, because it was *his* stuff that he couldn't cope with. Eventually I realized that AIDS doesn't mean death, and all the positive responses I'd been talking about could actually apply to me.

MARK (CANADA)

I was just beginning to spread my wings – I was twenty-one – so I had insisted that I went alone for the diagnosis, without my parents. We met at dinner that night. I don't know what I was expecting, but I knew that something was going to happen. My dad said what seemed the stupidest thing I'd ever heard – but when I look back it was probably the smartest thing anybody could have said. He said something like, 'Well, we'll deal with this like we've dealt with everything else, we'll get through it.' And I thought oh, thanks, Dad, that's brilliant, how philosophical of you!'

I thought it was completely naïve – 'We're going to get through it.' This was different, this was not what we'd had to deal with before, this was not a part of *me*. Haemophilia was part of me – I had no problems with it. I enjoyed being Mark, and part of Mark was having haemophilia. But this stupid AIDS thing was somebody else, wasn't me. I didn't have this when I came in here, I don't want it and to say we're going to get through this like we've got through everything else – you can forget it, this is different.

Some choose to remain silent to all but their closest friends.

PAVEL (CZECHOSLOVAKIA)

Well, I said to myself that I have to just stand it, everything alone. Nobody can help me and I just have to live with it. It wasn't for me something new, because I was more or less all the time alone. It was the same with homosexuality, because I didn't tell anybody about that.

I told it to only one person, a friend of mine living in Rome. More or less immediately, in a week. My best friend. I passed the first information by phone. These are not the things you should talk by phone, but it was necessary to spit it out. He's a strange person, very hard on himself and hard to others. He never showed a sorrow for me. It was a disappointment, a little bit. But he is that type of friend, he doesn't talk, he doesn't show anything.

He was a little bit angry at me, because he thought that it's due to some extravagant behaviour when I was travelling outside. Immediately as well he asked me how long I estimate I have it, because we had been living together, but we had no sexual contact for maybe five years. And actually he is not positive.

He was the only person who knew everything about me. I didn't talk to my family or to anybody else. I have some friends, but I haven't told anyone else, no one. I said to myself I have to absorb it alone.

And some tell no one at all.

ALICE (BOTSWANA)

The day I received a letter from the Red Cross informing me that my blood had been tested for four diseases, including AIDS, and one of them was positive, I nearly collapsed. But there were some friends in my room and I decided to put the letter away without saying anything. Since then I never told anybody. I am afraid to tell members of my family, because I don't know how they will react. I am even scared to tell my boyfriend. Since we met, he never had sex without a condom. I never asked him why – I just said thank God! I wouldn't have to ask him to wear a condom.

I never experienced anything negative from anyone, because nobody knows about my health. I would love my boyfriend to know, but I am afraid he might stop loving me. I hope I'll soon have the guts to tell my family members and him.

JOSHUA (ZAMBIA)

I worked as an untrained teacher for two years, while waiting to enter the seminary to be trained as a Catholic priest. I felt very fortunate to be accepted to start religious life. As some training is done abroad, I was told to undergo a medical test so that I could be allowed to go. Unfortunately, I was proved positive. I was told to discontinue priesthood life.

I was left without a job. Not even a reference to show that I had been with the religious men. I had no rest, but only turmoil. I was even afraid to meet relations and friends as I was certain they would ask me why I had come back from religious life.

I never went to anyone to be counselled. It was through reading books that gradually the fear started to go out from me. From time to time, the fear comes but I occupy myself with many things.

EARLY THOUGHTS

Many thoughts go through the mind on first learning the diagnosis. Some people immediately think they have a very short time to live.

REBECCA (ENGLAND)

I felt I was going to die very, very quickly. Certainly if you had asked me in December if I would still be alive now in September, I would have thought no. Although I was reasonably aware of HIV, I connected AIDS with imminent and swift death. In fact

I wasn't that informed, which I think is true of a lot of people. They don't realize that you have this long period of time of good health while having the virus.

MICHAEL (SOUTH AFRICA)

In December 1986, I collapsed and was taken to the local hospital. I had swollen glands and weight loss. The doctor in the casualty department examined me, asked a few questions and came up with her diagnosis. 'You have AIDS and have six months left to live'! It is difficult to explain my feelings. I was preparing myself for the Christmas season and now I had to prepare myself for my death – in six months' time.

I started planning my funeral, what songs were going to be played, who was coming and so forth. I still did not believe that I was no longer going to be on this place called earth after July 1987.

Some think of ending it all.

STEPHEN (UGANDA)

I was diagnosed HIV-positive in late 1988. When the news was disclosed to me, I thought of committing suicide straight away. Knowing that there was no cure for my problem, there was no longer any point in trying to live a little longer.

As I was deciding on the method to end my life, however, a second thought struck me: this problem is not mine alone, nor is it solely a national or regional problem but a global one. Somehow, somewhere, there must be people devoting much of their time to finding a solution to this threat to the whole human race. So it is possible that some time in the near future, although exactly when is not clear, a solution to this problem will be found.

Therefore I should struggle to live a little longer so that the near future might find me still alive and perhaps my normal health will be regained. I am now living in a state of hope, hoping for the near future to come soon so my normal life can be restored again.

There are also worries about being ill.

ERIK (SWEDEN)

I think one of my first questions, was, When am I going to get sick and am I going to get really sick really fast? What's going to happen today, tomorrow? I don't care about a year, five years, I don't care that I'm not going to live for ever, but how am I going to feel in the near future?

I didn't want to go through the pain, whatever it was. If I'm going to die anyway, kill me now, that's easier, I don't want to go through the pain.

Knowing about HIV also affects people's feelings about themselves. Feeling dirty is a common reaction.

IMRAT (MALAYSIA)

This doctor told my family that my cutlery should be kept separate. My clothes should be soaked overnight in bleach, to kill the virus. If I ever cooked I should wear gloves. I believed him – he was head physician, he should know what he's talking about.

I felt terrible, dirty. I felt that I have something in me that's dirty, that's running all through my body, through my blood. I'm not supposed to touch anything. I felt that if I touched my nieces and nephews I'd probably give them the infection. Because that is what the doctor told me, I should keep myself separate.

You feel frustrated, you feel why can't you be just like any other person. It's no good living any more, what the hell, why live any more?

SARAH (ENGLAND)

I just felt so filthy, really dirty. Unclean. I kept washing myself and having baths, thinking maybe I could wash it away.

It didn't happen to women, heterosexual women. Why did it happen to me? I must have done something really wrong. You don't think sensibly when you're told. I hated myself, I felt dreadful. I felt I must have deserved this, it was like it was my punishment. You hadn't been good enough in your life. It was like the wrath of God.

I was also frightened about dying – becoming ill and dying and not being able to look after my family. It was like a nightmare. You kept wanting to wake up. I felt 'This isn't real, I can't have this. I am so well and so fit and strong.' I just didn't believe it.

MARTIN (AUSTRALIA)

I felt that I was a biological hazard, that my body fluids were dangerous substances. That's what I felt – that my blood, my semen, even my tears were things that would put other people at risk. I still feel it a bit now.

You hear it's in a tear drop. How much worse can it get – you're not even allowed to grieve without some kind of contamination.

MARTHA (UGANDA)

Before I went to the clinic, I had poor health – constant pain, fever, stomach ache and leg pain. In 1989, I went to the AIDS clinic, where I met a counsellor who conducted me through intensive discussions on HIV and AIDS. I was tested and two weeks later I was told I was positive.

I couldn't believe it – it was really a shock. I tried to determine the route of infection and feared I would be called a prostitute.

There are also strong feelings of guilt or of being thought guilty.

WINSTON (CANADA)

I was just angry. I thought it was a punishment. I thought, somebody's punishing me for something I've done wrong, for my behaviour or whatever. I was an active drug user, I had sex. People I was hanging around with were living a fast life. I was into that at that time.

And I thought, why now? Why couldn't this thing wait another twenty years? Why not let me have my fun and be free?

My life was cut in half, everything was cut in half. I couldn't take things for granted any more. I had to start thinking of fighting to stay alive. I felt, I'm twenty-two and I haven't lived my life yet. That made me angry. And the fact I had, I thought, three years. How much can I do? How much living can I do until I'm twenty-five?

I felt, I've got a lot of living left to do. I have to fight to live. And as a black person, I thought this is only another struggle for me to go through. I believe the quicker that you deal with it, the better for you.

BEN (ENGLAND)

You feel that you've been singled out. Why me, why has it happened to me? You feel guilty because of promiscuity or whatever – all of these things that society has laid on you and you haven't come to terms with.

I had been married and I had two kids. I got divorced after discovering very late in life that I was gay. I'd ruined my ex-wife's life and I'd cut myself off from my kids for the sake of expressing my sexuality. For a few years, it seemed the best of worlds that men could at long last express their sexuality to each other. You could have sex with whoever you felt like with no holds barred. There was something very liberating in a deep way about sex in those days. If we wanted to make a long-term relationship we could, if we wanted it just to be for the sake of sex we could.

And then suddenly it seemed like God or whoever was saying, 'Aha, got you! You thought you were free!' It felt like one had been played a dirty trick on.

Some are primarily concerned about the effects for others.

ANGELA (SCOTLAND)

I never knew I was pregnant until three or four weeks after I had been diagnosed. The doctors wanted me to have an abortion, which I disagreed with. I was a Christian and I just said, 'Well, if God wants me to have this baby, He'll let me have it. And if He doesn't want me to have it, I'll have a miscarriage.' So I just took it from there. And I did have the baby. I think that was the easiest part of having the virus, because my concern was just for this baby.

Then, after I had the baby, every time I looked at her I just felt so guilty. She just looked so beautiful. I was told that she would probably die, I would probably die. And I said, 'What have I done? If she dies I'll never forgive myself.' But I was lucky, she did end up being negative at eighteen months.

MARTIN (AUSTRALIA)

I had one gay relationship in my early twenties – it wasn't really a relationship but a one-night stand. A lot of people like me, heterosexual men, have done this. I was getting bits of information about HIV and I was concerned about symptoms I had, so I decided to go and have the test. I told my wife and it wasn't any problem in our relationship.

But when I found out, it was a profound shock, an incredible shock. I didn't know anyone else who was HIV-positive. The first thing I thought was my wife would be infected. And I thought I probably had about two to three years to live.

I delayed telling her for a few days because she was going away to spend some time with her family. I thought this would be the last time she'd have with them without this thing. But I had told her I was going for the test and she knew from the tone of my voice that something was wrong. So I told her and she came back that night.

She had a test and that came back negative, which was really good. And she has remained so since.

And some think about how they acquired it.

KRISTINA (FINLAND)

I felt everything was lost, spoilt. No one else has HIV, I have. Why did I go with him? I should have known. I was accusing myself of being stupid, for not using condoms, for being with him.

I was bitter to him and I hated him. But then, you cannot hate somebody. He didn't know that he had it. But he could have been wiser. He'd been with other girls. I called him and he said it cannot be so, *he* cannot have it. Later, I called him again and said go to a doctor and he said OK. But after that, he has not contacted me.

MARY (ZIMBABWE)

After the positive result, I spent about three weeks without even talking to my husband. And then I asked him where he got that HIV from. He said he didn't know. I blamed him, because sometimes he slept outside with some girlfriend. Then he comes back during the morning. So I blamed him, he is the one who got it.

We quarrelled for a long time and then we just forget about it. I explain to him that we are a wife and husband and we have got HIV. We must endure things together. We must tell each other the disease you are suffering from rather than hide it. I should know what kind of disease I am suffering from. And then he say, 'I am so sorry, because I was afraid telling you that I am HIV-positive.' He had known for some two years.

Now, my husband and I, we are loving each other very much. We are closer, we are coming together, sorting our problems together, talking to each other. These things, it just happens in life. If I continue being against him, what does that help me?

PART THREE

Learning to
Live with
HIV and AIDS

From the moment people know that they are HIV-positive, many aspects of their day-to-day lives come into question – health, employment and how they spend their time. Some make quite radical changes in response; others continue much as before.

KEEPING HEALTHY

There is a very natural concern to seek out information about HIV and how to deal with it.

REBECCA (ENGLAND)

When I was diagnosed, I was one of these people who want to read everything and have as much information as possible. You have to know how to protect yourself, to feel informed about it and how you could give it to people.

I was very quick to get myself a social worker. She sent me all sorts of literature on diet, on any little minor problems that I might have, like thrush and skin conditions. She also sends a newsletter from America with all the most recent information about treatments available there.

There were also books. I didn't know that people lived for ten years after they contracted the virus. One had a lot of things to do for relaxation, positive affirmation, the sort of things you could say to yourself in the morning and little bits of meditation you could do. Which got me through that first month, dealing with panic.

You have to make very big decisions about treatment. Sometimes the medical profession can be a little bit cagey. They wait for you to ask, because they don't want to give you more information than you demand. But, of course, if you don't know what questions to ask, then you don't get the answers.

MARK (CANADA)

For a year or two after the diagnosis, I was given nothing from the haemophilia clinic, told nothing. Then, my curiosity began to build. On a number of occasions I asked how I was doing. 'How are you feeling?' I'd get. 'Well, I *feel* fine, but that's not the question. What does the *blood* say, what's going on in my body?' – 'Well, you're feeling fine, that's most important. See you in six months.'

Finally, my mum and I went in and were very clear that we expected to see this information – we'd take it and have it deciphered some place. So they gave us this series of T cell counts. I didn't know what these numbers were – 300, 200, 100, I didn't know what that meant. So we went to an HIV guy downtown and he had his own lab verify the numbers. He said, 'If those are your T cells, you should have been on AZT years ago.' That was a year and a half after I was diagnosed.

Things are a lot better now and I don't hold anybody really accountable. We all had a lot to deal with in those first years. This was a haemophiliac clinic that wasn't ready to deal with this death stuff. Everybody was slow in reacting.

PETER (USA)

It's a gradual process. I decided to go to conferences, that's how it all started. I heard things there I had never read, there were people there talking about the things you could do about this disease. Well, if you can extend your life for one day, maybe you can extend it for a year. If you can extend if for a year, why can't you extend it for ten years? All of a sudden, you see these things happening that are so positive.

I started a buyers club, to make sure that we have those things for sale that people with AIDS need. We sell additives, vitamins, unapproved drugs. I do anything to circumvent the shortage of my life. I believe I have the right to do so.

Some people become quite knowledgeable over time, and develop strong views about conventional and alternative therapies.

WINSTON (CANADA)

I'm healthy. I have no symptoms, nothing. I don't take medications – just one multivitamin a day. I stopped doing IV drug use, all the heavy stuff. I do alternative therapies, exercising. I swim a lot and I work out. I've been looking into Chinese medicines and homoeopaths. I will go on as long as I can without taking drugs like AZT.

A lot of people gave up, gave in to it. Talking with people who are long-term survivors made me stronger. It made me realize that those who fight determine how long they're going to live.

DANNY (NORTHERN IRELAND)

It's been like learning a new language, you know. Up until my diagnosis, 'CDs' meant compact discs, now they're CD4s and 'T cells' mean blood counts.

REBECCA (ENGLAND)

I take medication, AZT. I was advised to right from the beginning, because I had a very low blood count. But it took me a long time to accept that I needed to take a very toxic drug. I didn't want to put it in my body. And when I first started, I did feel quite ill. I felt nauseous and just totally exhausted all the time. But I thought, if I don't take it and I become ill, I'll never know whether I became ill because I didn't take it.

I've altered my lifestyle. I used to be a solid twenty-a-day cigarette smoker and now I'm an occasional roll up smoker. I barely drink at all any more. And I have changed my diet. It's important for people with HIV to avoid meat, because so many of these parasites and food poisonings come from meat dishes. I make sure that I get a healthy diet and all the nutrition I can possibly get. I take vitamin supplements.

I have massages and shiatsu, a form of acupressure, which is brilliant. It's an Eastern practice, quite a spiritual thing, but for me – not being a very spiritual person – it is more the hour of the week where I 'indulge'. It's simply taking time for myself. It's the one time when I truly am able to relax.

Stress is a big factor when you're diagnosed HIV. It's very difficult to live with this virus. You are under a lot of stress, often you can't talk to people about it. So shiatsu's really helpful.

ERIK (SWEDEN)

I didn't change my lifestyle much, I can't really say I did. I'm careful, I try to avoid infections. But I still eat junk food and I exercise less today than I did.

I stayed healthy, with just minor infections, until August 1989 when I discovered a lump on my neck. I was admitted to hospital and treated as any cancer patient. I was treated very well, but it was terrible, because I felt that my body had let me down. I said to myself, I have been fighting so hard to stay healthy and now my body does this to me. I was scared, of course, but mainly I tried not give in to the disease. I took an active part in my treatment and the examinations. The doctors encouraged that, but I was in hospital for four months. That was a long time.

I trust my body, I know my body does what it can for me; if I help it a little, my body will do everything I ask it to.

Positive thinking is needed, guided imagining. I can encourage myself. If you believe in yourself, if you're strong in your identity, then you can affect your whole system. I have seen it happen with my patients. If I can encourage them to work – not just with their body but with their whole system – with me as a caretaker, I can heal them, we can heal each other.

IMRAT (MALAYSIA)

I'm not seeing my first doctor any more. Instead of doing any good, he was damaging me more with valiums. I now have a lady doctor, who has a wide experience with AIDS work. She doesn't put me on any kind of drugs or pills. It's *words* which I think are really important.

Words make you feel wanted. She makes me feel that she cares, she gives a damn about *me*. It's really great, it's more important than having vitamin pills or the 'nervous wreck' pills they were giving to me. I have not got any major infections, nothing. It's been five years, not on any special kind of diet. No drugs, nothing.

I lead a normal life. I still take alcohol, even though some people say it's bad, I still do the same things I did before.

I don't think that having HIV means that you should change your life – change your diet, stop smoking, stop drinking, you should stop having sex and all that. I think that's rubbish. Why should you change being what you are? I think that being positive is what it's all about.

In some parts of the world, there is also witchcraft.

JONATHAN (UGANDA)

My father was a polygamous man with three wives, including my mother. My mother divorced and we stayed together. She started to think that I had been bewitched by the wife currently at home. She started taking me to native doctors. They asked for goats, chickens and money, telling us that the ancestors were annoyed that the other wife wants to kill me, because I am the natural heir to my father. To clear my way from all these bad spirits, we had to present all these things.

I was given local herbs which one can't imagine. Late at night, the doctor would take me out to bathe in rotten eggs spread in very cold water. One day I was put in a hole covered in banana leaves and soil, with firewood put on top and set on fire for twenty minutes. I could feel the heat on top. It was supposed to burn away the evil spirits. I was cut with razors all over my body and smeared with herbs to drive away the evil spirits inside me.

We went on doing this for a complete month, until I mentioned to my mother that this was a hospital matter.

It can take a long time to adjust.

ANGELA (SCOTLAND)

I hardly used to drink before I was diagnosed. And then I just went through a period of drinking all the time. Especially at weekends. Eventually it got to the stage where it was every night. It just started to be a part of the routine in my life.

I started to feel really ill, not physically but mentally. I couldn't eat and was letting myself go. I was getting thinner and thinner.

I went through four times of really wanting to commit suicide. But there was that wee thing – the kids. I got to the stage where I couldn't even stand the kids touching me or talking to me – I just thought myself that bad. It was as if I just wanted them to stop loving me, so that I could make it easier for them as well.

Now, I just try and live as normal as I can. I watch what I'm eating. I do still take alcohol, but not very often. I still smoke, but I've never touched drugs since I stopped.

Some have to come to terms with looking different.

ERIK (SWEDEN)

I have fungi on my toenails, it's not contagious, but I feel that it looks disgusting. It's not dirty, but it's the feeling I have inside. I love to walk barefooted in the summer, but now I feel ashamed to do that, because people will look at my feet and say, 'What is that?'

I also have venereal warts, they're very common among gays, so it shouldn't really be a problem. But I'm a little bit ashamed of those things, I don't want to be a show. And if I would have a KS spot somewhere, I would never take off my t-shirt again.

I can't really explain it, I just know that it's not very nice. I'm a bit ashamed that I actually feel that way, because what is a spot on the stomach or the chest?

Drug trials can become part of a person's life.

PAUL (USA)

My experience with HIV began in 1988. I came down with PCP [pneumonia] and was consequently diagnosed with AIDS. Like a lot of people, I had never been tested and had no idea that I was positive.

After recovering from the PCP, I needed to start anti-retroviral and PCP prophylaxis treatment. My doctor suggested that I look into clinical trials. I took his advice and enrolled in a trial; I am the only surviving patient on study at this site.

In November, I was diagnosed with peripheral CMV retinitis in my right eye. After much deliberation, I decided to seek experimental treatment to maintain my present life: laser surgery and oral DHPG. The laser surgery was the easy part. My opthalmologist had experience with the procedure and encouraged me to try it. The theory is to burn a wall to prevent the spread of infection. I had this in December 1990 and to date there has been no spread of infection.

I also needed to treat the retinitis with DHPG. Syntex research is conducting a number of trials for this, using both oral and/or intravenous therapy DHPG. I chose to go on the Phase One trial, so that I would get the oral drug, and succeeded in becoming the last person in the US to enter that trial. My retinitis has remained stable. Only one other subject has remained on the drug for this long.

Because of the willingness of both research groups to work

together, I have been able to remain on both clinical trials and to receive the best possible follow-up I can.

MARK (CANADA)

I was on AZT for a year and a half. I quit it, went on a ddI/AZT trial and I quit that a month ago. I just had enough of the guinea pig thing, of tests, of appointments. And putting something in my body that I had no idea what it was doing.

I take Chinese medicine. I see a Chinese doctor and he just gives you herbs. They've been at it for 100,000 years or so, so I figure they must know something.

SOMEONE TO TALK TO

Being diagnosed with HIV can lead to great isolation. It helps to meet others in the same situation and many people become involved in support groups of one kind or another.

WINSTON (CANADA)

I thought, I can't deal with this alone. I have to tell somebody. There have to be other people there for me. I moved to stay with a relative. We were quite close, so I told her the situation and she said, 'Well, there's a support group and maybe you should check into it.'

It took me about a month to build up the courage to do that. It was a matter of being visible. Seen going into an AIDS organization. People are going to assume. I went to see these people called Body Positive. It was once a week for about ten weeks. It was very informative, each week was structured, they dealt with issues of bereavement, dying, all the medical issues and how do you tell partners and when do you tell partners and family and friends. It was really good. Also I met other men who are in my same boat.

MARTIN (AUSTRALIA)

Eventually, it took about a month I suppose, I found a support group. It was incredibly supportive and I used to go once a week. That was really important for me.

It started the process of normalizing it. Up until that point it was like you didn't know what to do.

What was hard was that there was nothing for my wife at all. There were no other women whom we knew of in the same position, no other couples, and she was very isolated. It's difficult to encapsulate how that felt. It felt very isolating, we'd been cut off from the norm. You'd suddenly been taken outside what you were used to.

SARAH (ENGLAND)

When the woman at the clinic said, 'Would you like to meet another woman with HIV?' and gave me her phone number, I couldn't wait to get home. At five o'clock, I dialled the number and we were talking for maybe two hours, non-stop. It was incredible, I was on a real high.

As soon as I met her, it just changed my life. I realized I hadn't done anything wrong, I wasn't a criminal. We've become firm friends. We have good laughs which is what – when you're HIV – you tend to lose. We had cuddles, she was great – vibrant, alive and full of fun. An amazing character.

We've formed a women's group. We used to go to a mixed group, but we found we were looking after the gay men there, listening to their problems and not getting anything out of it ourselves. First, we were only two women, but gradually other women were put in touch and we started a group just for women.

We used to hold it in people's houses, but we found that the person that was hosting it would be making tea and not getting involved. So now we have it in a building where we use a room. It's really good, it's going really well.

I can talk about problems that have happened. Not just to do with HIV, but the children or if I've not been well. Just supporting each other, having good fun, having a laugh.

BEN (ENGLAND)

Last weekend, I went to the national conference of Body Positive groups in Britain. It's a very liberating experience to be with two hundred other people who are HIV-positive. You don't have to hide anything, you don't have to worry, you can talk about anything – symptoms, how you feel, what drugs you're on, the way that you deal with problems.

By working for AIDS agencies and going to AIDS and HIV conferences, I'm probably happier than I've been since I've known I've had HIV. I'm less isolated, because I know that I'm not the only person in this situation.

ROSA (URUGUAY)

After my husband died, I started to fight with other HIV/AIDS-affected friends for our own lives and dignity. We started visiting people in hospital whom doctors and nurses were preparing to face death. We started to give them affection and we became nearer to them in both physical and spiritual ways. Showing no fears, we started to touch each other, tell each other our own stories and share our feelings, fears, doubts and hopes. This began to give our lives a new meaning and different values. Lives that many people thought would be extinguishing very soon. Instead, many patients recovered sufficiently to leave hospital.

Some are helped more by a one-to-one relationship.

IMRAT (MALAYSIA)

I tried to commit suicide twice. You feel useless, you're just going to be a rotting vegetable in bed. You're not going to contribute anything. Instead, you are just going to be a burden to your family.

I was not working. Free time means you have nothing to think about – you think about yourself, what you're suffering, what AIDS is.

The greatest need was to be able to talk, to relate to someone how you feel. I had my family, but family is a family sort of thing. You need someone who's gay, who knows about AIDS. Someone who can lead me, shine some light here and there, what you should do and what you should not do to remain healthy.

Finally, I said to myself I need to talk to someone about it. We had an organization, a gay organization which also dealt with AIDS issues. I made an arrangement to meet a counsellor and this guy sort of brought me out. He made me realize that you are not dirty, you are just another person in the street. You should not feel different. There are a lot of things that you can do.

DAVID (ENGLAND)

I went into therapy, still am in it. That's been very important, to try and look at the deeper issues. It took me a while to set that up. And to build up a support network that was real. I thrashed around a bit; because I had been involved in setting it up for others, it was quite hard to receive it for myself. That continues to be a tension in my life. But it's something I'm learning.

I had this depression. All they did at the clinic was put me on anti-depressants, dreadful things. They nearly blew my head off and made me feel dreadful, for weeks I could hardly speak. Then I laid them off and the depression came back. And I thought, there must be other ways of dealing with this. I spoke to someone who was an adviser and he introduced the idea of therapy and said that he would find some money to pay for it which is what happened.

It's helped tremendously. I don't get anything like the depression I used to.

DAILY LIFE

People often wonder how they would spend their time if they were faced with a life-threatening disease. Some undertake drastic changes in their day-to-day lives.

BEN (ENGLAND)

One thought one's life had come to an end. Surely it's the same as anybody who'd been given a terminal diagnosis, which is what it felt like in those days. If you've got a short time to live, you go through all kinds of things. You contemplate suicide, because you don't want to go through the pain and the distress of the actual disease.

I didn't know who to turn to for advice, I was just shocked. And there was little point in doing anything, since the main thing seemed to be that I was going to die in very short order. The information in those days was very garbled, but I must have read somewhere that the life expectancy was eighteen months. I certainly had that figure in my head.

I thought, well, I'll just sell up and go to all these places that I'd always wanted to. I didn't tell anybody. I was completely on my own. I left my job and sold the flat and went travelling round the world – thinking that I'd find a nice quiet corner to die in somewhere. It didn't happen, of course.

Eighteen months later I found myself abroad, having spent all my money and not dead and no sign of being dead. So I got a job and had five very fruitful years teaching before I did get ill.

HELEEN (HOLLAND)

I've been riding all my life, horses. I am very specialized in horses. I worked with horses. I did everything – I can shoe them, I break them in, I give lessons, I had a horse riding school.

After the diagnosis, I went to where I was working. I had a

very good contract, but I just said I was leaving the country. I was going, I didn't want to carry on with my very good contract. I thought I was going to die in a year, why should I go and build up something?

After three days, the doctor phoned and said, 'We talked with the hospital. I shouldn't worry about anything, there is nothing happening yet.' That was after I already ruined everything. Because I talked to everybody and everybody knew I was leaving.

I thought I was going to die in a year. And then, later, I found out I had more years. I lost a lot of money by not knowing that straight away. I should have gone on with the project I had with horses.

MARK (CANADA)

I wanted to go back to the way I used to be, when I was just a kid like everybody else. All of a sudden my life had changed and I wanted to go back. I remember seeing this ad in the paper saying 'childcare work with summer camp component'. It was working with children with severe emotional and behavioural problems.

It was anything but summer camp. These kids had been really messed around their whole life. And you were their parents, the closest thing they've ever had to a parent. They have an amazing way of making you feel their pain – and in the process making you feel stuff that's going on in your life. About a year into it, I just completely broke down. And that was when I really realized what HIV was.

I just understood what it meant about life and death. And that it was time to stop ignoring it. It was releasing a lot of that first year of denial. It just came crashing down, it was like a cocoon I was coming out of.

The people there were very supportive, it was great. They allowed me, in a healthy way, to get over it and get on with it. I didn't know at first how it would affect my employment, I'd only told them about my haemophilia, not the HIV. I wanted the job. In fact, when they saw 'haemophilia', they figured that one day they would be dealing with HIV as well. So, they knew, although I hadn't told them.

Shortly after, I left, because I knew that I had to get on with being involved in the HIV thing.

Others slowly adjust plans in the light of their infection.

REBECCA (ENGLAND)

I was a student of primary education, a mature student. I was diagnosed at the end of my first term. I finished the year and then decided that all the reasons that I'd wanted to go into primary education didn't apply any more. I'd actually wanted to teach in the developing world and that isn't possible, because I need constant treatment. And I'm at risk from infection.

I'm trying to be more open about my HIV. People like us, who are infected, hide our status. We have to because of the stigmas attached, because of the prejudice, because of fear of our homes and our jobs and our families. As a primary school teacher, I would not be able to do that. The subject of children is very emotive and if parents found out, they would probably take their children away.

I'm now concentrating on English literature. And basically just seeing a degree as a valuable achievement in itself. It took me a long time to get to university from school, seven years, so now my ambition is to get my degree. Just to say I've got it. That's two years away and if I'm still around, then I'll make a decision about where I go from there.

ROBERTO (MEXICO)

It was September 1986. It was not only an earthquake in the earth, it was an earthquake in myself. A personal earthquake. All my life changed – I lost my apartment, I had a lot of problems with some friends, I had a lot of problems with my family, I was in trouble.

I decided to return to my psychotherapy. I was in therapy two years more. My life changed slowly. I can say that the better years of my life are probably these five years. It was not a dramatic reaction for me. Because I had seven years just working with myself, psychological examination of myself.

In the beginning, my employer was very good, asking how I am and sending my money, my salary complete. I was the director and they spoke with me and said, 'Probably it would be good that you change and not be a director. You can be a professor only.' It was good, because a director has a lot of responsibility, much stress. I said okay, I accept.

And now I am working in the school, I have a very good place. I am a good professor, I know and I love my work. I love to teach, it's some fascinating experience for me. And I am working in psychotherapy with my friends. It's another work that I love very much. I think I am a privileged man.

JENNIFER (UGANDA)

I had five babies – three died and two are still alive. My husband divorced me. I was diagnosed HIV-positive when I had my fifth baby.

I started attending the day centre for comfort because my baby had died. I learned tailoring, handicrafts, sharing experiences with existing clients and helping where needed. The whole sense of death from AIDS disappeared; I made up my mind to plan for the future of my children. At the same time, I have benefited much from yoga exercises, which relax the body and mind and reduce drug consumption for minor infections. I am now the yoga instructor.

Through counselling, the AIDS organization discovered that we HIV-positive mothers have a common financial problem. A club was formed to meet our needs and from discussions, income-generating activities were suggested. These are handicrafts, poultry farming and breadmaking. So far, we have started with the handicrafts and a small scale project.

DAVID (ENGLAND)

I trained to be an Anglican priest. I wanted to be a priest at a very early age. I think it was part of my struggle with authority, to prove that a working class boy could break down the barriers of the institution of the Church of England. But I also was aware at a very early age that sexually I was very different.

I discovered that I could earn my living outside being a parish priest. I have a lot of skills that I hadn't realized and that I've been able to sharpen. It feels like I've been created for this part in my life from the beginning – that my priesthood and my sexuality and my virus are all part of the plan. It's taken the virus in my own bloodstream to enable me actually to address those issues. And to let go of the things that I've hung on to. That sounds neat and tidy, it's not like that at all. But that's an element in the journey. Somewhere in all this, I've found an identity that allows me to be articulate.

And a few decide to continue very much as before.

PAVEL (CZECHOSLOVAKIA)

My job is sometimes tiring, because it's very irregular, sometimes I am working from the morning up to night. I just had to answer this question to myself, if I am capable enough to proceed in this kind of job. I consulted a doctor friend of mine – he knows how I am living – he recommended me to take care, but to continue. Because he preferred the psychological calm.

I think that's important, to continue as before.

One reaction is to undertake work with AIDS organizations.

MARTIN (AUSTRALIA)

I couldn't think of a way of actually dealing with this, with being HIV-positive. Do I go and have counselling? Do I do alternative therapies? My way of dealing with it was to get involved with people who are HIV. My job was producing information, doing public work with health care.

A guy I worked with was one of the few people in Australia who was open. It was his example that made me want to go on television and say things and be public. I've been public as a person with HIV in Australia – radio, TV and newspapers. To try and challenge that image, to make it easier for people who are HIV-positive to know there are other people around. Also to challenge people's attitudes, to do something about the bigotry that's around.

BEN (ENGLAND)

I do a lot of training. I go round to hospitals and anybody that will have us. We talk about HIV and AIDS and ask them what they think about it. They always think that somebody who's got it is going to look like a skeleton and be on their last legs. We talk about it and then I say, 'Okay, well look at me, I've got AIDS.' And, of course, I look perfectly fit. It shocks them to think that I've had AIDS for eighteen months and I still look totally fit, fitter than most men of forty-six, I would say.

My priority now is to stay alive and do what I can to give something back to the community, to help to educate about HIV and AIDS and to support people who need support.

WINSTON (CANADA)

I do volunteer work. I got involved with the buddy system, being a buddy with people who have full blown AIDS and are really sick. I had people close to me die in my arms. That was tough, because that was seeing my own mortality and saying it's a matter of time, my time will come. This could be me at some time down the line.

But the pain that they were suffering, they had to deal with themselves. I wanted to help, but you have to do that alone. After years with the disease, this is something I've come to realize. Those who are not infected, like my family, the pain they feel is pain I cannot touch. And that hurts. I can see that people are afraid, but that's just the reality of the disease.

Being a buddy made me strong. I'm fortunate to be doing this and it made me more determined to give more, to do more for others. The more I do, the more I get rewards. No matter how painful it is.

I'm starting work as an AIDS co-ordinator in a community complex. That will be part-time, which I'm happy about, because I need something else, distractions. I don't want to make AIDS my whole life, it's not my whole life.

I was doing work for nothing, sitting on diverse boards. Everyone expects that I should go on doing it for nothing. And I thought, here I was sitting in conferences and speaking with consultants – consultants who knew nothing – and they were paying them $900 dollars and giving me two bus tickets, thank you. I had to scream at them, 'I can't do this for nothing. I want to do this because I believe in it and it has to be done. But you have to take care of me, too.'

I threaten a lot of people, being visible. In my city, I am the only black man who is visible in the media and who's putting a face to this. So there's a political issue, because most people of colour who are out there go underground.

ELIZABETH (UGANDA)

I became a counsellor in a missionary hospital almost immediately, when I was told I was HIV-positive. I felt it was my duty to help in counselling others, since I was more enlightened. I wanted to help patients, especially as far as spiritual life is concerned. If any were afraid to die, that was not the end of life. There is life after death. I wanted to give them that comfort and assurance, that if they forgot about their disease and looked upon their Creator, that will lead them to eternal life.

LUCIA (ITALY)

I am a lesbian and was a drug addict for about six years, from the age of twelve. I got off drugs six years ago. Just then, I found out about being HIV-positive. It was very hard at the beginning, but I kept doing what I had planned for myself: get off drugs and start a new life.

I moved to London where I lived for more than a year with my girlfriend. I got in touch with some HIV-positive organizations for the first time. Back in Rome, I started to work for various AIDS organizations, and in January 1991, founded Lesbians and AIDS, a group of women who felt the need for a clear voice in AIDS regarding our health and social issues. We are strong and we are fighting for our rights.

Some have real financial problems.

MARY (ZIMBABWE)

My husband lost his job. He didn't tell them he was HIV. But he left his card in the office and someone came and opened the drawer and saw it. He gave it to the boss, who said, 'Oh, are you HIV-positive? You'd better go. We don't employ people who are HIV-positive, because they are going to give others the virus.' He is looking for work now for three years.

Money is very difficult. Even my children, they don't eat properly. It is very difficult. Children who are HIV-positive need something which is good, which gives proteins and vitamins. So if you don't give them that, it's really very hard. Where are you going to get that food from? In Zimbabwe, food is very expensive, so it's terrible.

It is hard to manage because if I fell sick or my children fell sick, there is no way we can go to see the doctor or the hospital, the clinic. It is very hard for us.

ANGELA (SCOTLAND)

I've just started applying for grants and things last year, because I never knew you could get anything. I met a welfare rights worker and she did all that kind of work for me and I did get a grant.

I was just living on benefits before, getting loans for things I needed. Then I discovered that I was allowed £12 ($22) extra for a disability premium. And she put in for back money that I never knew I was entitled to, which helped with the house. It makes quite a bit of difference. I have had my struggles with money, but we get by.

STEPHEN (UGANDA)

My monthly salary can barely support me and my family for just a week. God knows how I have managed to survive up to now. Some of my family members have started falling off. My dear wife died two weeks ago, leaving me with four children – three of school age and an eleven-month-old – to look after.

WINSTON (CANADA)

This year, I went away for Christmas and my place was broken into, so I lost a lot of stuff. I went to an organization for emergency funds and they said, 'You're very healthy! What needs could *you* have?' I want people to realize there are people who look healthy like me, who are infected. I may be smiling and healthy right now, but that doesn't mean I don't have needs. I need a job, we all need that security of paying the rent.

EXPERIENCES OF REJECTION AND ISOLATION

People with HIV do not experience rejection every day. But a number have had their lives touched by some incident, involving a sense of rejection or stigma of some kind.

BEN (ENGLAND)

I decided I wanted to try and rejoin the church that I grew up in after many years' absence. So I took confirmation classes and I thought I had a good relationship with my church. I was perfectly open with them. One day I offered to work in their coffee bar as a volunteer and at first they said yes. And then they realized – 'Oh my God, you're HIV-positive. No, you can't work in our coffee bar.'

This kind of reaction is very hurtful, because you realize they think of you as a leper, as some kind of unclean person that shouldn't be let near their precious cups and saucers. It makes you angry.

I left the church and went to another where I just keep that part of myself private. Because if you tell some people they're just not able to cope with it.

PIERRE (BELGIUM)

I've known for five years that I am infected. They didn't talk about HIV then – I was a 'not totally AIDS' patient.

I was fired because of being HIV. I put this in the open, through the TV, radio and the papers, the political parties and union organizations. They all told me that it wasn't right, but they didn't do anything. Even worse, the union was going along with the factory. Here in Belgium it is difficult to find HIV or AIDS patients who want to co-operate, because the fear of discrimination is so big.

I busied myself with preventive work. I loved doing that, it started a whole new life for me. It didn't make the discrimination disappear, but I could stand it better. But the pain stays.

PHILIP (ENGLAND)

Recently, my wife was in a large London teaching hospital, pregnant with twins (now born). The hospital knew my antibody status. My wife was barrier nursed, given meals on paper plates, ignored often, and there were all sorts of detergents in big bowls in the room. The doctors washed their hands before shaking hers. At least five doctors came in while I was there and asked questions about how I felt living with HIV.

A giant *'Infection'* was written above her name. She was asked to use a separate toilet from the other women, which had a red

'*Control of Infection*' notice on it. She was miserable, frightened and scared for her children.

I realized what was happening and complained. The attitude was, 'Oh, we know HIV isn't contagious, but we must follow our old guidelines.'

Our babies are alive and doing well.

LUCIA (ITALY)

I am angry. Because now exists serious information. I don't understand the mentality. Last week when my friend died, people didn't want his clothes, because he died of AIDS. It's stupid because the virus is dead. I think it's only because it's AIDS. It's homosexual or drug use – it's not the virus, it's the background of people with HIV.

JOSIE (ENGLAND)

Unknown to myself, my Spanish partner had dabbled with drugs. Shortly before the birth of our son, he explained everything about his teenage life. I wasn't particularly worried. After all, he seemed so together and normal.

We moved to England. My partner, being in a foreign country, became less confident and the old habit returned. He was very devious and I didn't realize for several months. When I eventually did discover what was happening, I was horrified. But I supported him and slowly weaned him off the heroin.

In 1987, he became ill and was admitted to hospital. The doctors gave him an HIV test (without his consent) and promptly told him he was HIV-positive. He was in total shock. He never told his family. I was the only person he told. I tried to be supportive, but he refused to talk about it and every week he would have some illness or another. He became very withdrawn and depressed.

Over the following few months, he meticulously planned his own death. He told the doctors he couldn't sleep, so they prescribed him sleeping tablets. One morning he drank half a bottle of wine, took some pills and saying, 'Goodbye, Beautiful' to me, quite normally went out of the front door and threw himself under a car.

I was treated appallingly by the local police. They came to my house to tell me what had happened and they were very sympathetic, until – well, I was in shock – I told them he was HIV-positive. I told them, in order to safeguard other people. What a mistake. Their attitude to me and my son changed.

The next day, I found that my confidential conversation with the chief inspector was all over the local papers. I had the press knocking at my door, hounding the neighbours, trying to take photographs of myself and my son. They even went to my son's school.

I had to leave our home and move to another city.

Many feel isolated and alone.

MARY (ZIMBABWE)

People in Zimbabwe, they are really against people who are HIV-positive or suffering from AIDS. Even if you teach about AIDS, they say that you are the one who has got AIDS. They don't understand that being HIV-positive doesn't mean that you have AIDS.

So when I knew that I was HIV-positive, I sat down and started thinking about it. Who am I going to tell? What if my parents came to know or my friends – what are they going to say about me? They would say, 'You've got AIDS, we don't want to greet you' or 'We don't want to share some juice with you, because you are HIV-positive.' People are saying it is spread by shaking hands, using the same toilets, kissing, using the same cups or plates.

I wrote a letter to Zimbabwe officials to help me with my children and they replied that we don't have people who are HIV-positive in Zimbabwe. And I asked, 'My husband is not working, what can I do to make my children survive?' They say, 'It's your own fault, we can't help you.'

RASHID (MOROCCO)

I am one of those who owe everything to their family. That is
the way I have been raised. We are manipulated from birth to
adulthood. You may do whatever you want if you are studying
overseas, but once you are back, you have got to get back to
the classical track: job, marriage, children and parents twice
a week.

The problem with HIV and AIDS is the fear. You cannot afford
to be identified as AIDS people, you just have to take the same bus
with the others, while you know that you are not going in the same
direction. You just keep smiling when frustration makes you cry
inside yourself.

There is something worse than AIDS in this country – pressure.
It cuts off your ambitions and, at some points, all interest in life.
AIDS people need sometimes more help and support than others.
If we meet only incomprehension and rejection, what interest in
life is left to us? We are less ready than anyone else to cope with
these problems.

ANGELA (SCOTLAND)

Hiding it from people was my biggest problem. I can remember
one day, my husband's mum was getting a cup of tea and she
offered me another cup. She asked, 'Oh, what cup were you
using?' And then I was thinking, does she know? None of us
had told her and I was worrying, does she suspect?

I had to face that people were going to suspect me, because
they know my past situation using drugs. Going into a pub one
night with a friend, a man did turn around and say, 'What are
you doing, palling about with her? She's used drugs, she's got
AIDS.' But they were just surmising, they didn't know. You had
to go through a lot.

I desperately wanted to let it out, but because of fear –
protection of my family – I couldn't say anything. I've got a
big fear of rejection.

I told one person and that was through drink. That was the

biggest mistake I made in my life. It went everywhere after that, everybody got to know. My husband blamed me and I got a healthy doing for it. He kicked me, I'm sure he was trying to kill me. I landed up in hospital with a broken jaw.

I got to the stage then that I was scared to go out. Going into the shopping centre was my biggest worry. Because that's where you bumped into everybody you knew. And you got looks. Twice I heard at the back of me, 'That's *her* that's got AIDS.'

When I was pregnant, my brother said, 'Are you fine? Have you been checked for hepatitis or anything like that?' I just stared at him and the fear came back – if I tell him he might reject me. He was my closest family, my brother, and I was scared. I said, 'No, I'm fine, I've had hepatitis.'

I found out later that he was trying to tell me about *him* – he was positive. I thought he had escaped it and he thought I had escaped it. He committed suicide, because he couldn't handle it. If he had known I was positive, it would have been a great help. He never had anybody he could talk to. He felt he had no life.

Some just have a general fear of never knowing when their diagnosis will be a problem.

DAVID (ENGLAND)

It happened on holiday in Greece. I fell over, my nose was bleeding and it was very bloody, I'd fallen off a wall late at night – I'd had a drink. All the people that were with us, we'd never met them before, were coming around with blood everywhere. And my partner said, 'Don't get involved in the blood, because David's HIV-positive.' And that was quite a shock to us both. They were a bit stunned, but they were fine in the end.

I suspect there's a whole area of people that avoid me like the plague. There was an article in the paper about me, about my diagnosis and all that. I see lots of the young people and they all wave. But there must be lots of others who perhaps turn the other way or who say terrible things. But I'm not aware of that.

And some experience 'sympathetic' reactions.

MARK (CANADA)

I talk a lot about 'buckets'. There's a bucket for the 'faggots' and a bucket for the 'drug users' and a bucket for 'the people who got it through blood'. They're all treated very differently by society. The homosexuals just 'deserve exactly what they got', that's what society tells us. The drug users are 'no good to us anyway, so it's better off they're dead'. And the people with haemophilia: 'It's too bad, what happened to them.'

A lot of that really annoyed me, from day one. I was no different from anybody else. Nobody asked for this virus, nobody wanted it in their life. I'm no different. Everybody else, when they find out their status, asks the same questions I did – what did I do to deserve this? It just twists me when somebody says, 'You were exposed through blood – oh, I'm so sorry.' I'd rather I got stroked with the same brush as the others.

PART FOUR

Relationships

In the many joys and trials of life, it is relationships with others which generally sustain people. All such relationships are put to the test by the introduction of a life-threatening disease. People have to learn new ways of coping with each other, make judgements about what can be talked about and when, and generally think about what will happen when they are no longer there.

PARTNERS

Relationships with existing partners change.

MARTIN (AUSTRALIA)

I have incredible admiration for my wife, deep love. I just think I'm really lucky. After we got involved in AIDS, we met some couples in a similar position and quite a few relationships didn't survive the diagnosis. Ours did and I think that's due to her, really. She's a very strong person, I can't really say more than I love her very deeply.

The diagnosis put a strain on our relationship, it was difficult for a while. My wife has always been incredibly supportive. She wasn't frightened from the beginning, didn't believe the myths about HIV and AIDS. We'd always been fairly honest with each other about what we'd done, so that made it easier to talk, but it was hard for her.

She needed to talk about her grief. I think her need was to talk about her fear for me. And the fact that we had been advised not to have children, which we'd both wanted. That's been an ongoing problem for both of us. We found a support group where she could come along, a mixed group, gay and straight. For the first time she was able to talk about what she was feeling. They were really nice about having her there.

One of my concerns is that she doesn't invest so much in me, that if I get sick and die it leaves her with a big gap in her life. That's really difficult. She has an emotional investment in me, obviously, we're in a relationship.

And for a long time, I was concerned about infecting her. That was a major problem, I felt so infectious and contaminated. I still feel every time we have sex I'm putting her at risk.

Underneath it all, she still thinks about having kids. There's nothing I can do about it, nothing. So it's trying to find things in her life to substitute for kids, which isn't easy. There's the dilemma of her having a life that's her own.

MARY (ZIMBABWE)

Before, my husband was moving from one place to another looking for girlfriends. But he is now good, he is a good husband. I feel happy that he has changed.

I didn't understand before. In the first days, I was a girl so I ignored AIDS. It affected people who – or prostitutes. Then after I got married, I started to think about AIDS, maybe I am going to be the one who is going to suffer from AIDS. Because you can't trust your husband, he can have many girlfriends outside and then he will come into you, you love each other, so you never know.

We don't want another baby. My husband is saying that if you are HIV-positive, if you become pregnant, maybe your baby will be suffering from AIDS. Who is going to care for the baby? So I decided not to have another baby at all. I have got family planning tablets. We can love each other.

Some new relationships, begun with full knowledge of the diagnosis, are very strong.

DAVID (ENGLAND)

I met my partner two and a half years ago; we've lived together for two years. He has AIDS – he nearly died twice before I met him. He's ten years younger than me. We were like teenagers, we just went bang and love, over the coffee table at the local centre.

It's been marvellous to do all the things we've always wanted to do and enjoy them with each other. Every day is a new gift – for me, but particularly for him who really has been near death twice. He's one of the most powerful characters I know, charismatic and loving, so it's good.

I was a very lonely person all my life. The relationship with him is a very domestic supporting one, which I really appreciate. The loneliness I used to feel has gone.

REBECCA (ENGLAND)

I have a partner who is not HIV-positive, who I met after I was diagnosed. We've lived together for about three months now and I've known him for about eight months.

I felt very guilty about even thinking I could go into a relationship. But I got a lot of support from my women's group and I went ahead and started seeing him. I told him very quickly – I didn't intend to, but I felt I was drawing him into something that he had a right to know about. Which was the fact that I had a life-threatening illness and I'd had it for some time.

I was fortunate in that he'd known a woman who'd had HIV before. He hadn't been involved with her, but he was very informed of the risks. He went away and thought about it – that's what I wanted him to do. He said his major concern was not about contracting the virus, but getting involved with somebody who might die. But he had decided that whatever time we had together would be worth it. And he wanted to be a part of my life until that happened.

I felt an immense sense of relief. And, I suppose, a little bit of gratitude that he could still see me as a human being who was worth loving. You lose a lot of confidence in yourself when you're diagnosed, you wonder whether you are still a worthwhile person to love. He's the person who has helped me the most. He loves me and he's not frightened by me.

It has become less and less of an issue in our relationship. Of course, we had to talk right from the beginning about sex and how we felt about each other. We've always been very open and able to talk about how we feel.

I work very hard to make sure that he still has space to feel sorry for himself, because I think he does feel a bit apprehensive. And he feels very cheated. He's fallen in love with somebody for the first time – and that person may well be taken away from him. I think there has to be room in our relationship for him to have those feelings. Without me saying, 'How come *you* feel that, when *I'm* the one who's going to die?'

We have a perfectly normal sex life. I made a decision early on that if he felt uncomfortable with any kind of sexual contact with me, it was his responsibility to tell me and we would deal with it. I had enough to deal with without worrying about whether I was going to infect this man. We have protected sex with a condom, we avoid oral sex, but apart from that I don't think there's anything that changes our sexual relationship at all.

He has tests every three months and he was negative at the last one. I am confident that he will stay negative, because it's actually quite a hard virus to get if you understand how to protect yourself.

I made a decision not to have children. It was very hard, I still get upset about it. Pregnancy is very stressful on your immune system. But more, my decision not to have a child was that I want to be alive for the whole of that child's life. That's a responsibility I would have to that child. And the chances of that would not be very good at the moment. It's not a constant pain, but it's another one of those losses.

Some people are very conscious of the special needs of their partners.

HELEEN (HOLLAND)

I've just got married. I think it would be very important for my husband to speak with other heterosexuals, who are negative and who are living with a positive person. Because that's something very difficult.

I have been always very open and I have now to respect him. He has to go through all those mills, to get used to it and not feel ashamed any more for living with somebody who is HIV-positive. That's a very difficult thing for him. He loves me, but he doesn't dare to tell his friends.

But people living with HIV and AIDS can experience considerable difficulties in their relationships, including direct rejection.

KRISTINA (FINLAND)

I'm afraid every time when I fall in love with somebody, I start thinking, can this lead to marriage? Or what's going to happen when this gets so far that I need to tell him? That maybe he's going to reject me and say, 'Oh no, Kristina, we cannot continue any more.' I have faced that twice already.

The first time I was dating, I told him that I had been tested and it might be positive. He didn't believe it, but I said, 'It's true, you have to believe it, you have to face the fact.' He has been with me anyway, he has been my friend and a bit more than friends. But when I asked, 'Can you marry me?' he said, no. Because he wants children, he doesn't want to use always condoms. And he's afraid that he's got it, too.

Then another man I told, we had really good fun. I couldn't tell him face-to-face, so I wrote him a letter. And he called me, he said that he had been crying reading my letter. He said also that he cannot think of continuing with me, because he doesn't want to fall in love with a girl he knows she's going to die. I said everybody's going to die. He said also that he doesn't want to use condoms always. I didn't tell him that I was angry, but I was angry at him.

I've been crying, but I'm still friends with both of them.

JUAN (COLOMBIA)

I am thirty-two years old and the father of a very beautiful daughter, aged seventeen months. I found out that I had AIDS when she was only three months old. Even though I was discreet about being gay, my wife was furious and threw me out, saying,

'I can't go on living with a homosexual.' It seemed to be more traumatic for her to know that I was gay than to know I had AIDS and would by all accounts soon be dead.

The only person I got help from was my sister.

ANGELA (SCOTLAND)

It was the first guy in my life that I thought was easy-going, never violent. The relationship started off good. Then one night, he never used a condom; he said, 'I can't stand the things, I'm not using them any more.' And I thought, how do I get out of this one? But I just couldn't tell him, I was so scared of being rejected again. So I let the relationship go on and on.

Then I started to feel guilty about not using condoms. I got myself into a right state, low and depressed. I really wanted to tell him, but I was so scared of the reaction. This went on for months. I took the guilt on myself – if anything bad happens to this guy, I'm going to feel responsible.

Then I thought he's got to feel guilty as well, he's the one that wanted not to use condoms. We had the odd discussion. He did ask me why did I have leaflets, did I have AIDS? I said no, only I was interested in working with people with HIV. He said, 'Are you, like me, scared to go and get tested?' and I answered 'Well, aye.' I didn't know what to say.

I'm glad I never told him. He was scared to get tested, so obviously he didn't want to know. In the end, I knew that it was never going to work, because he just didn't want any responsibility.

I'll never go through anything like that again. I'll always make sure to bring up the HIV.

It can become a time when people want closer relationships.

ROBERTO (MEXICO)

I changed my relation with boys. For fifteen years, I preferred the fun, the gay bars and so on. Now, no. It is not something good for me, a lot of people. But I had no one person being close to me. And each day, each month, each year,

I feel the necessity to be in love, to speak with someone only.

And suddenly it's true and I am in love now for two months. I am in love with another positive boy and it's a very interesting and a fascinating relationship for me. We met in a group of HIV-positive people. We are very close friends, but our sexuality is very small. Our relationship is principally the affection, the tenderness. I think it is the kind of relationship that I need now – not a very passionate one. For me, it's very good and I think for him also.

It has nothing to do with HIV and AIDS. I think it's to not hurt each other and take the time you need. If you care about each other, why rush? I feel much more secure if I can find a safety with the other person first and then develop a sex life after that. I've changed, I put other things in the relationship.

I want a loving, a caring, an understanding, a trusting relationship – those qualities and then other qualities.

SARAH (ENGLAND)

I'd love to have another relationship. But I don't look at men, I'm really frightened about getting involved with anybody else. It's rejection. Fear of being rejected and of infection, of passing the virus on. Because I know how to have safe sex. I know you can't pass it on through kissing. But it's actually knowing that and then getting to the next stage.

I've lost a lot of confidence. So I'm a bit scared.

And then there's coping with sex, including whether and how to tell potential sexual partners.

WINSTON (CANADA)

Abstinence was an issue. The whole idea of practising safe sex – when you're young, it's not what you want to hear. So I just got turned off it, no sex.

After two years, I thought this is not realistic, this doesn't work for me. It was a matter of telling people who I wanted to get close with. It wasn't easy. I had to make my own decisions and I had to deal with the reactions, negative or positive. I didn't know how to say it – did you tell them after the fact or did you tell them before? It was rejection that I was afraid of, but you have to tell them.

I use humour. Humour always works. It makes it easier for them to deal with it and to talk about it.

I had to learn about safe sex and to practise it. You find ways of pleasing yourself without penetration. That was tough. And the fact of wearing condoms – you find excuses, they don't fit, they ruin the sensation and the feeling and stuff like that. But then, I have to protect others. It's about responsibility – if I don't take that responsibility, who's going to?

You come to realize who likes you and who doesn't. It's a heavy thing to deal with. People stop touching you and all these little silly things – they don't want to kiss you, don't want to hold you.

Some were quite supportive, closer. Sex changed. Down to the fact of being close to them was important, for me and for them.

MARK (CANADA)

I continued to have relationships with women. I never had a bad reaction. I'm not the kind of guy that five weeks into a relationship says, 'I have something to tell you.' I don't know how people do that. HIV is such a huge part of my life, I can't sit down for five minutes without breaching that topic. What else is there to talk about?

I made a clear commitment to myself that I would never put anybody at risk. And I would define risk within each new relationship – between myself and my partner, we would decide what risk was. For each relationship, it would probably be a bit different. But I have my own line that I will never cross. I will never have unprotected sex, without a condom, with anyone. That's where I draw my line.

I make sure that this person has all the information and that they've digested it and understood it and then we talk about what we feel is safe, safer, risky, riskiest.

DANNY (NORTHERN IRELAND)

I enjoy sex – always have and always will do.

I remember meeting someone who was obviously very drawn sexually to me, as I was to him. It got to the stage of who's going back where tonight. We were going back to his place and I said, 'Before we go any further, let's talk limits, safe sex. If there's going to be any screwing of any description, condoms.' I'm the kind of person that likes things up front, generally. He said, 'Well, I'm clean.' I said, 'I'm sorry. Once upon a time I was in your position, I thought the same as you, but the reality is that I am HIV-positive.'

After that, it became very clear that nobody was going anywhere that night.

FERNANDO (BRAZIL)

I tried to suppress my sexuality because of fear and guilt. It was hard, I had many psychosomatic illnesses, culminating in two motorcycle accidents. Then I built up a monogamous relationship with an extremely handsome Afro-Brazilian man and we had a wonderful time for three years. He died last March, one month after he discovered his virus state. I found I was HIV-positive last May.

My biggest concern now is about love and sex. I need to have close physical contact with somebody. It feels like I am twenty-one again, when I first began to be homosexual. When I go to a gay place, it is as if it is the first time. The sense of something forbidden, fearful. And guilt comes out every time. The latest reports suggesting that oral sex and simple wet kisses may also infect really limit the possibilities of spontaneous pleasure.

It becomes more difficult when people (mostly people who are not HIV-positive) say that I should stop my sexual life. This is pure suicide. How can someone in a good state of mind interfere in a basic human right?

PARENTS

Some people have easy relationships with their parents, sharing their hopes and fears readily with them. But many find this relationship full of tensions. Telling parents of a life-threatening disease is clearly very difficult. First, there is the matter of finding the right time.

SARAH (ENGLAND)

My father had been asking me for a long time. He knows me really well and he'd be sat in the kitchen and he'd say, 'What's wrong? What's wrong, my love? What are you worrying about?' And I said, 'I'm fine, it's nothing.' I just wanted to tell them so much. I really wanted their love, their unconditional love. It doesn't matter the state of me or what I'd done or anything, that was what I wanted.

I'd told my brother. I've always been very close to him, so I told him first. He was really upset, he kept saying, 'I wish it was me, you haven't done anything to deserve this.' Then he couldn't face my parents because he knew this about me. Three weeks after I told him, I phoned him up after work and said, 'Tonight's the night.' And he said, 'Good, do it.'

We got home and my mother was in bed and my father – I always used to go in and chat with them – I went in and sat on the side of the bed. My dad said, 'What is it? What's wrong?' And I just couldn't say it, it was just so hard. My dad held my hand and he just said, 'Look, come on, nothing can be that bad.' So I sort of blurted it out: 'I'm HIV-positive.' And they just cried and held me and asked if the children had the virus.

It was very strange. My dad's got a really dry sense of humour and we were laughing, crying, then he put his arms around me and said, 'All I can say is, thank God you're not pregnant!' Because usually I go in and say, 'Dad, I'm pregnant again.' My mum just held on to me and said, 'I won't let you die, we're all going to fight this together.' She was really strong.

They were just wonderful. So supportive. They were cuddling me and holding me – when you're HIV you don't get touched – it was just so important. It was what I needed, to have somebody. I needed to talk and talk.

I always was close to all my family. The thing that has changed is that they're much more open about their problems. Whereas before, they wouldn't tell me things, they confide in me – to do with business and emotionally. So we're all much more open about everything.

And my brother's bought a bigger house, so that if anything happens to me there's a home for my two younger children. After he did it, he said, 'There's always those rooms for anybody.' I was really touched.

Some parents are very supportive.

DAVID (ENGLAND)

I think the most difficult thing was telling my mother. She lived with me at the time. I was terribly depressed, she'd been away for a bit and came home and – I don't know why – I just burst into tears. She said, 'What is it?' and I started to tell her and she said, 'You're trying to tell me you're HIV-positive, aren't you, dear?'

She's eighty-three years old, she's great. That's been marvellous. I realized that it's not just about HIV, it's about my relationship with my mother. And everything about me.

She's very proud of me. She talks about it all the time. She's learnt a lot too. She comes to all our meetings. She can't hear very well, but last week we had about sixty people there and she said, 'I just love to be in the midst of you all, because I've never felt such love.' That's great. I'm sure she must think in the quietness of her heart, 'What the hell's going on? My gay son.' She's got all that as well.

IMRAT (MALAYSIA)

I had very good support from my family. They said, 'You are part of the family, you are the son in the family, why should you be treated as a different person?' They make me think I am one of them, that I am still important in the family. And they make me feel that it's okay to have what I have, there's nothing wrong in it. It's just another disease that not many people know about.

I did feel very good that my family understands me, because if *they* didn't understand me, who else *could*? It makes me feel wanted, appreciated, even though I had the infection. To know that your family's not rejecting you, but they're supporting you in every way they can.

My family knew I was gay only when I told them I had HIV. They had to adjust to that. They did not talk about it, they did not ask me any questions about it. I told my mum and she said that it doesn't matter. She said, 'I always suspected that you were gay, because you always had calls from guys and letters from men and none from girls.' I had a very bad fight with my brother-in-law, who said he cannot accept that I'm gay, he wants to change me to straight. But it doesn't really matter, because my immediate family understands it.

But relations with parents can be very strained.

WINSTON (CANADA)

What didn't work out was the family thing. My immediate family was in another city. I told them, the ones who I thought I was close to, and to my dismay I wasn't. They isolated me and said, stay out of their life. That was the harsh reality. They weren't close to me at all. I accepted that.

It took me seven years to tell my parents. I believe that some things are better unsaid. I live with it. I don't want to deal with them, because they can't deal with what I have. That's not my issue, that's their issue.

ROBERTO (MEXICO)

With my parents, is a different reaction. My mother loves me very, very much. Nevertheless, five years ago she spoke with me about my homosexuality. She is in a religion, very fundamentalist with the Bible, and their position is that homosexuality is not acceptable at all. And my mother spoke with me in a very hard attitude that you are doing some things terrible. And my reaction was more hard, so there were some difficulties with her.

But in April, I spoke with her and I said, 'I'm sick, I am sick with AIDS. I don't know what will happen with me in the next year.' I said, 'Finally I will die, I don't know how long time.' And my mother she responds with a very very – She did not change her idea, but she is a mother. Well, she took a lot of care with me. My father is a little bit different, because he's a seventy-year-old man, very sick. At the same time when I was sick, he almost died. My house, it was like a hospital. Later, my father was better and my mother spoke with him. And it's a problem. My father and me never talk about the situation, never.

REBECCA (ENGLAND)

I am relatively close to my family. I didn't feel that I could pretend that something very dramatic hadn't happened. I wasn't intending to tell my mother until after Christmas because I didn't want to ruin Christmas for everybody, but within an hour of coming to see me she knew that something devastating had happened. Although I was fighting to keep control over my feelings, I simply wasn't the same person I had been two weeks before.

My father didn't want me to tell anybody. That was his initial reaction. I think he was ashamed. Very worried about how I would be treated if people found out. I think they feel if I had to get some life-threatening illness, perhaps I could have got a slightly more socially acceptable one for their age group. Like cancer.

Sometimes that's the story that's given. It makes me very annoyed, that they're not honest about it to people who are close to them. I have HIV and I'm not ashamed of having it.

Many parents are undoubtedly very isolated in their knowledge.

MARTIN (AUSTRALIA)

My mother finds it really difficult. She's probably frightened I'm going to die and she just doesn't want to have to deal with it. We're still working that one out. I've spent some time with her recently and it's not easy for her to talk about. I want to take it gently.

She's in a very isolated position. She's in a small town and she's a bit anxious about people finding out. She doesn't have anybody else she can talk to. It's really hard for her.

It's not just about AIDS or HIV, it's about our relationship. We were very close, my father died when I was young and our family was very close. I've tried to keep that closeness, but she's got older and I've changed and so there's that as well to deal with. I reckon it complicates things. I don't know how I can comfort my mum. Because I can't say it's going to be all right. If I'm honest, I don't know.

Some people with HIV live with terrible reactions from family.

PRUDENCE (BOTSWANA)

My husband died in 1988 and left me with five children, six months to ten years. The baby nearly died. With him dead and me infected, life was surely not on my side.

My parents-in-law wanted me to divide every little asset in the house, from plates and pans to the bed. A few days after the burial, my father-in-law was looking to sell my sewing machine. Since some sympathizers were still around, I told them and he cooled down for a few days.

I had a set of oxen and a plough and one day, while I was at the hospital, I came home to find the children telling me 'many uncles and grandpa came for the oxen. They said they are taking them to keep somewhere.' I discovered where and why they were taken. If I kept digging with the plough, I would be very rich food-wise and I wouldn't run away. So I should starve with my children, face real hardship and that would make me run away, leaving them to remove whatever they wanted. But I remained strong and people helped me with my work and, thank God, I now have something to feed the poor kids.

Then they wanted to sell a bull, again without my knowledge. Soon after, they wanted to sell one of the three pieces of land which according to my late husband, was to be for his three sons. This was too much for me. I had to apply for a letter of administration. The case was heard, but up to now it has never been judged. I have tried to consult my lawyer but all in vain. I was really stranded. Thank God, since the court day, they have not sold much, as they also fear a bit. One of my bulls was stolen and I believe they are the ones, for some evidence was proved. I believe the money was used to bribe the magistrate to delay the whole thing.

However, to their dismay, I am still well and strong. So what they now want to do is to poison me. They have so far tried two people, both of whom came to tell me. This has given me a lot of worries. Because God made money and money can make men mad. One day they may land on someone ready for the money.

Some never tell their parents.

KRISTINA (FINLAND)

I didn't tell my family. No. I was thinking of my mother, how it would affect her. I think she doesn't even know about AIDS and HIV. I'm afraid how they will react. I'm afraid that they will start cleaning the dishes. I think they should know how it's transmitted, but I'm not able to tell them. I don't want to do that right now.

And I feel that my mother would have said to me, 'Oh, Kristina, why you did that mistake again? Always you are making mistakes.' I'm also afraid that my older sister would say that.

Somehow, I feel that if I tell them, it would bring us closer to each other. But yet I haven't done it. Maybe I have to take care of myself now, go through the crisis and then tell them.

BEN (ENGLAND)

I had a severe case of pneumonia and all of my friends quickly realized what was happening. People put two and two together, they know that you're a gay man and you've got pneumonia. It doesn't take great intellect to put two and two together. Some people have had the same information and chosen not to make that connection. I've respected that. My parents chose to do that.

My mother just died and I'm glad she died without knowing, because I don't consider that the anxiety would have helped her. My dad seems to continue to choose not to make that connection, so that's fine. He's of a different generation. It's hurtful, because one would like to have support, but he's old himself. I have to give him support on his terms, not on my terms. He doesn't want to have to deal with this at some level. That's his choice. I find my support in other ways.

MARY (ZIMBABWE)

I did not tell my parents. If I tell them, they will be against my husband, because they love me. So I decided not to tell them. I am going to tell them when I develop AIDS, not now. If I tell them now, maybe they are going to hang themselves.

I fell into an AIDS rumour, that I'm suffering from AIDS. My parents spoke to my husband, saying, 'Are you the one who give my daughter AIDS?' He said, 'Who told you that?'

And we took them to the doctor and they were assured that I am not HIV-positive. The doctor felt that if he tells them, there will be a war between my parents and my husband. Which is not good.

My sister, who I am living with, does not know. No one. Neither my relatives nor my friends, they don't know about it, about myself. The only person who should know that I'm HIV-positive is my husband. But it's very hard for me not to tell other people.

CHILDREN

Some people have children when HIV or AIDS enters their lives. Telling them is the most difficult of all.

ELIZABETH (UGANDA)

Elizabeth's children were aged fifteen to twenty-five when their father died; it was at that time that she told them she was also HIV-positive.

I didn't know how to give the message to my children. It took me about two days to think about it and I asked the Creator to give me a way to tell my children. I gained courage one evening, called all of them together in the living room. Still my heart was pumping, trying to gain courage because I didn't know what their reactions would be.

It was the only opportunity now that they were all on holiday. I didn't want to tell some and leave others. I asked them what they thought killed their dad. All of them didn't know, they couldn't suspect their father to have such a disease, such a gentleman whom they loved so much.

When their father was in hospital, one of my sons was anxious to see what AIDS patients looked like. They were kept together in one ward and everybody knew it. My husband was in the ward of top civil servants. Now, this boy stole himself away and went down to that AIDS ward. When he came back, I asked him where he had been, he told me with a smile that he had gone to have a look at AIDS patients. In my heart, I said if only you knew you had a case to look at, you wouldn't have bothered going down. But of course, I didn't tell him.

So the children didn't know what killed their dad. When I told them, it was a shock in their lives. And, I said, as a result of that, I am also positive. Some of them moved away, two girls remained and one of them said, 'I suspected, but I had no facts.' I thought it was my duty to talk to them further and comfort them, give them assurance. I had done my duty. I breathed a sigh of relief, because I did care about their reactions. I said to myself, 'I have done it at last. If anything happens to me, they are aware.'

One thing I have noticed is that they seem to be scared of marriage. It has affected them. My daughter who is twenty-five would very much love to get married – all her life she wanted a home. But that feeling has faded away, because she's scared. She thinks men are not trustworthy, she wonders who she can trust as a husband. And she thinks that all – most – boys are affected, especially in our country. So she has declared that she is not going to get married until this thing clears away. How is she going to live? She's not alone. We have had a number of young people like that. It's very hard.

WINSTON (CANADA)

I've got three kids, sixteen, twelve and nine. They've been tested and they're not positive. They are very supportive. They're very aware, I'm very tuned in with them.

My eldest son took it hard, because he's going through a thing where one of his classmates is dying of AIDS. So when he's seeing that, he sees me. Daddy's going to die and that's a big fear to him. We die anyway, so I explain that to him and how I feel. It took him a while to get close to me, he kept his distance. Then he came around and I showed him how to use condoms and put them on and I talk frankly with him on stuff like that.

SARAH (ENGLAND)

My daughters are twenty, eleven and nine, my son's eighteen. The little ones don't know. They know Mummy's not well, they know something's wrong with me, because I have to have my blood taken.

I told my son when he was sixteen. That was the hardest thing I ever had to do in my life – telling him that I've got a potential death threat. He became a little boy, he hugged me – he'd stopped doing that – and he just said, 'Who will look after us?'

I said, 'I'm not going anywhere yet, I want to stay well. And I need your support.' And then afterwards, he'd keep touching my hair or doing things he would never consider before. Like putting the rubbish out or if I had loads of shopping, carrying it for me and things like that.

PETER (USA)

I decided to come out of the closet with my disease. I wasn't so concerned about the effect on me, the question was what would happen to my son?

I have two sons, one was living with me. I didn't find it difficult to tell him about the HIV. I found it much more difficult to tell him that I was gay. I thought telling about the HIV might be worse, but at the same time it's only me that makes a big deal out of it. They do not.

And I'm very healthy, I can show them that I'm a healthy person with HIV. So maybe they'll learn about the fact that you don't have to be the person that lies in the hospital, with tubes sticking out of every orifice.

My son's friends and I had already become very close, because they suspected it. At that time, there was AIDS material lying everywhere, so frequently they would ask questions about AIDS or they would ask questions about sex. So we had already become very intimate.

They made it very clear to me that I had a message to give. And that message was much more important than the possibility of them being hurt by me being open. Of course, I was thrilled about that. I thought it was a very mature attitude on their part. I don't know what I would have done if they had said no, because eventually I would have come out of the closet in any case.

Perhaps even harder is how to handle small children who are HIV-positive themselves.

MARY (ZIMBABWE)

My little boy, just two years eleven months, I can't believe that he is HIV-positive. I just keep it as a secret. I will tell him when he's older. You've got to look after him. If a child who is HIV-positive is just there for five years and then he dies, I just feel he should do what he wants. My other baby died only three months old.

FRIENDS

Raising the subject of HIV can bring friends closer together, although not invariably so.

SARAH (ENGLAND)

I only told any friends this year. I've got three whom I've known all my life, since I was three years old. We see each other once a week, and they tell me all their problems. I always thought I was deceiving them, but I was also wary of losing their friendship.

One night, we were all sat together and one told me that she'd been wetting the bed for twenty years. That was a real thing for her to say, she really opened up about it all.

And then – I don't know, it just happened – I said, 'Well, actually, I've got something to tell you, I'm – ' I couldn't say it, but eventually I did and they have been absolutely fantastic. They just were so sad that I hadn't told them before.

IMRAT (MALAYSIA)

I had a lot of friends, a big circle of friends. I was not sure how they would accept HIV. When they asked what was the illness I had, I always told them it's leukaemia. I felt that was the closest thing I could link to. That word just slipped off my tongue and I just had to carry on and on.

But they were a very concerned bunch. One of them called the hospital and gave my name and said if he ever needs a supply of blood, do please call back. The doctor said, 'He's not suffering from leukaemia, he has AIDS.'

We are very close knit, so word got around. That changed a lot of things. They stopped coming to my house, no phone calls, except for maybe three or four. I felt rejected – rejected and disappointed. I felt they did not understand me, they were not my friends all this while. I was disappointed and frustrated with them.

Later, I told other friends. If you tell them you have HIV, you have to tell them you are gay. That's harder, because they always felt you are straight. But I just opened up. It took them by surprise, they said, 'How come you don't act like a girl? You smoke, you drink, you haven't tried to seduce us.' My reply was, 'You are straight, I respect you for that. That is what I want from you, to respect me for what I am.' They understood that.

I think I've been closer to them. In fact, they have met my lover now and whenever they're going out anywhere, they invite both of us along. Which shows that they really understand me in a positive way.

ANGELA (SCOTLAND)

We were friends for two years, before we even knew about each other. It was really weird that night. We'd been drinking and I just turned round and said, 'What do you feel about people with HIV?' Her response was really good in what she was saying, so I said, 'Well, I'm HIV.' And, well, she just started laughing and she went, 'So am I!'

We really helped each other; since we've known, we go to a lot of places. We're not true friends, she's a lot younger than me, she's like a companion really. HIV makes us close, but you couldn't say there was a really true friendship.

REBECCA (ENGLAND)

I told one friend right at the beginning, who completely went to pieces and couldn't cope with it at all. That actually put me off telling people for quite some time. It was a male friend, whom I had been very close to. The thing is, people in their twenties, one of the big issues is not HIV itself but death. It brings up a lot of stuff in people about their feelings about their own death.

And also whether they'll be able to watch you become ill and die. I think this was what absolutely terrified my friend. He would say to me, 'I don't know what to say to you, I don't know what to do.' And I would say, I want to be treated as normal. But it was very difficult for him initially.

ERIK (SWEDEN)

My friends are my family. I would rather call my best friend if I'm taken ill. There's a guy, he's older than I am and he's also HIV-positive. We have known each other for many years now and we have become best friends. When I was in hospital, I would not have survived without him, because he was always there for me.

I have never felt a stranger among others. I've always been welcome. And most people that know about my HIV status, at first maybe they're a bit reserved, but when they see that I am still the same old me, it changes. They feel – most of them – that it's okay, we can live with this. Most people are just sad for me, they don't want to see me die. We're friends and they don't want to lose me.

If relationships changed in any way, they became closer. I don't think my friends did anything specific, they were just there.

PART FIVE

*Reflections on
Living with
HIV and AIDS*

People living with HIV and AIDS, not surprisingly, give a lot of thought to how they should live.

LIVING ONE DAY AT A TIME

A common reaction is to live for the present, taking each day as it comes.

PAVEL (CZECHOSLOVAKIA)

I just live very much the present time. I am conscious that my time is quite short – limited or restricted. I can't make real projects for the future, because for me it seems to be a little bit nonsense. For example, you hear news from the television about the year 2000 or something and for me, well, maybe I won't be here.

I just try to be realistic, I just say to myself listen, it's like that. We are here temporary, everybody. And it's all relative, if you are dead at the age of eighty or fourteen or forty. It's nature, it happens like that.

I'm a bit fatalist – it may be typical for the people from Eastern countries. Because we were quite a lot manipulated. I don't want to exaggerate, because in my country the liberty was not so suppressed. But we were less used to our own independence, to our own responsibility. I became a bit fatalist. I took things as a fact of my destiny.

SARAH (ENGLAND)

I don't look too far to the future. I just live a day at a time.

I'm much more careful about who I choose to be with. Every day has to be very special. I wake up and think, today's going to be a good day, so I want to be with people I like.

And simple things, like waking up and seeing the sunshine. And looking at flowers, seasons changing. And thinking, God, I've made it – here we are coming up to Christmas! I don't want anything major out of life. I just want to enjoy my children and my family. Just simple things, making a nice meal and having fun. Life's precious. Well, it is for us all. But in a way we've got the privilege of being able to prepare for our death. And being able to enjoy our life, however long we're going to be alive.

There is often a concern not to waste time.

PETER (USA)

Time is of the essence. For many years, I dealt with that sentence in my business and suddenly it became a reality to me. Because time *is* of the essence. Every day has a new meaning for me.

If I had to live my life over again, I cannot think of anything that I would do different – and that includes contracting the illness. Because it has meant a lot of personal growth to me and I think the quality of one's life is superior to the quantity of it. To live a long and empty life is the last thing that I would want to suffer.

I find myself much less judgemental, because I've gotten to know the world a little bit better. On the other hand, I have become much more angry, because there is so much callousness that should not be around. I can get very outspoken to those who tread on people like ourselves, who desperately need help.

On an AIDS vigil in Washington DC a few years ago, I walked past the archives building. And there was inscribed in stone: 'Everlasting vigilance is the only road to liberty.' I thought, what an odd thing to be engraved in stone. But the more I thought about it, all I wanted was what is on that stone – equal access to treatment, universal health care, no more discrimination, a little bit of love and a lot of compassion for all those that have a disease.

MARK (CANADA)

One of the first things I found was that I had no time for bullshit any more. I had no time for people that I don't have a real desire to have in my life. Like one girl that I'd known in high school who heard through the paper and called me up and wanted to hang out. We hadn't talked in ten years and we never had a connection to begin with, so what's this about?

And other things, just stuff in my life that was a waste of time as I saw it. Time is the most precious commodity I own and for me to spend one moment of it doing something that doesn't please me is a waste.

Many express a love of being alive and the need to appreciate life to the full.

ROBERTO (MEXICO)

I think that I am privileged because I work, I am in love, I am travelling, I have very good friends, I have money, I have not problems with my health. I feel myself well.

In the life, I am very much an observer. I like to be looking – the people, the things. I have a marvellous relationship with one of my nephews, I love him very much. And to see him growing each day, it's marvellous for me.

I think that life is a marvellous gift, just thinking and learning about the marvellous universe.

IMRAT (MALAYSIA)

My outlook towards life has changed. You don't take life for granted any more.

Life is valuable not only for yourself. You also want to do something for other people. I feel more giving and sharing. It makes me feel wanted all over again. Everything has changed.

I feel now that life is more valuable, despite HIV. I'm lucky to be still here, to be able to live and to do the things that I want to do. Before I was diagnosed, I couldn't be bothered with life. You take everything for granted. Now, everything you do, you appreciate it more. Even to the minor things, like if you go into the garden and plant a rose. It's going to grow one day, then it flowers. You appreciate life around you.

I think having HIV is great. It has changed my life. I have no regrets. If I did not have HIV, I would not have changed my life. I would not have this positive outlook, I wouldn't be caring about people or about myself. I think I am very lucky having HIV. Not everyone can get it.

BORIS (BULGARIA)

It is now eleven years that I have been living with my boyfriend. We are a happy couple. When one year ago we discovered we both had the HIV virus, my first reaction was natural and human – almost unbearable grief and sorrow for our young lives, about the future which did not exist any more, about all the beauty of the world we could never ever contemplate together.

For more than one year, I have been preparing myself for the great encounter with the nothingness. On the surface, my life didn't change at all. Even more, my family life visibly improved and now is almost perfect. Evidently, the tragedy helped us to resolve one of the most essential problems of mankind – to learn how to live together. What a pity it is so late.

Some suggest that one effect of having HIV is that they have become more serious.

REBECCA (ENGLAND)

I think the most dramatic change has been I've lost a little bit of my youth, my joy. Everything's a bit more serious now.

But I'm stronger. When you're HIV-positive, you say, 'Well, I cope with HIV, I can certainly cope with that.' You've had to build up a real strength, but I wonder whether sometimes that strength cuts you off from people. You have to be much more in control of your emotions.

You live with every day. You have to sort out your feelings about the fact that your life is going to come to an end. Most young people think, 'I'll worry about that later.'

I've appreciated the value of having people around who love you and of loving people. Everything becomes more poignant, an experience that you need to appreciate. You haven't got for ever any more.

KRISTINA (FINLAND)

I believe I have changed. There are both good and bad sides. The bad sides are that I feel I am more serious. Because you are not able to have fun, to enjoy life. Always you are thinking only problems, problems, problems. How bad the world is, how many problems there are and they cannot be solved.

But I've changed in that I can now live more in this moment. That I shouldn't look backwards any more, but go straight ahead and live this moment. Every person should live in this moment and not in the past. To be enjoying life, not giving up.

Not everyone sorts out their life easily.

ERIK (SWEDEN)

I went into a state of shock, like a glass bowl, and I stayed in there. It was very fragile but I could keep it as a protection. I don't think I really tried to deal with it. Two years later, I had a problem at work. I felt that I lost control of everything. This little bulb burst and things that I hadn't really dealt with came up.

I was afraid of getting ill, of course, and I was afraid of dying. I realized I'm young, twenty years of age, and I didn't want to die. I'd just started my life, just started to find the real me. I had friends who loved me, I loved them. Life was starting to be easy.

Before, I'd had troubles. My mother died and there was a personal family crisis. I had a difficult time discovering I was gay. So I felt that I had a reward now, I have endured my life and now I got the reward. And suddenly this terrible ghost came and takes this away.

Also the insecureness of what's going to happen – when is it going to happen? To never know, if you go to sleep tonight, how will you wake up tomorrow?

UMBERTO (ITALY)

In 1989, I moved to Ireland. I only had a few friends and little knowledge of the local social network. In December, I was diagnosed as HIV-positive. Around the same time, the news reached me of the death of four friends in London. I experienced depression, anger and guilt not knowing what to do with it all.

My partner tried to be supportive, but I felt very isolated. I refused to contact the local AIDS helpline or to go for counselling. I got involved in setting up a company and for about eight months my life became just work and nothing else. In retrospect, this was my way of avoiding the issue – proving to myself that being HIV was not bothering me. In December 1990, our company went out of business and I found myself unemployed, physically unwell and emotionally stressed.

One day I happened to watch 'Stories from the Quilt' on TV. I cried – at last something from the outside mirrored my feelings. Even though they were from America, I felt the presence of those people in my life. It was a thread to get hold of. So I went to the opening ceremony in Cork of the Irish Quilt tour. Again I cried and I had to leave the hall as I found it difficult to express my feelings among so many people.

The realization then hit me of what I had been doing to myself – self-discrimination. I was gay and HIV-positive and this was to me like being at the very bottom of the ladder. I had spent day after day feeling dirty, guilty, worthless and fearful, and I was now finally starting to find my freedom. My life was opening, there was a future to live for.

Living with HIV is certainly not easy; the only way to live positively with it is to have lots of courage and share the challenge.

MICHAEL (SOUTH AFRICA)

My life has been like an emotional roller coaster, the only problem being that I cannot get off. Sometimes it is very difficult to remain on a high, but I endure because, after a low, there has to be another high. I still get angry with the disease, because it is going to carry on infecting people. And I get angry at people who ignore education and still believe that it cannot happen to them!

I do not think that a person ever comes to terms with this disease. Sometimes I feel as if I am an actor, wearing different masks all the time – when I am at work, when I am with family and friends. It is scary to think what will happen when the final curtain comes down.

To me, it is not important what stage of the disease I am, what is important is that I am alive, willing to live and learn for today. There is no guarantee that *anyone* will be here tomorrow. Therefore it is vitally important to live for today. It is sad that at the time a person most needs support it may be withdrawn because of the nature of the disease.

THE ROLE OF SPIRITUALITY

A diagnosis of HIV is a time to review the spiritual aspects of life.

PETER (USA)

I'm very much a spiritual person, but I'm not a religious person. I would find it insulting to myself to belong to any organized religious movement. The Church has been absolutely conspicuous by its absence in this whole epidemic and does not deserve my presence.

However, spiritually I think I have grown a lot more. I believe that there is something there that guides me along. And if I was made in God's image, then I am completely part of what God's image is all about. I do not have to go to a building to celebrate that I'm part of God.

I very much believe that there is some hereafter. And in whichever shape it will come, it will be a surprise. Since all of us are going through that surprise, it couldn't possibly be bad, because nothing goes without a purpose in this world.

BEN (ENGLAND)

My relationship to Christianity has always been shaky, which is why I left the Church when I was about twelve. I've always maintained a spiritual dimension, though. Most of my friends turned out to be Christians in a very understated way, and I realized that they had a kind of spirituality that I related to.

But I'm definitely very sceptical about a lot of the Church's teaching, and I sometimes run a mile at the things I hear from the pulpit. I'm just trying to come to terms with that. I'm hoping to make some contact with some Christians that are not judgemental.

My relationship to God is simply that I think it is helpful to suppose that there is something outside oneself to which one gives thanks. When I was abroad, I frequently found myself in a place on a mountain or by the seaside, and I would just give thanks for all of this. It's just grace, it's just a gift of grace.

Thanks for still being here. Thanks for the sunshine, the flowers and friends and all of the good things in life. Thanks even for having HIV, because it's brought me to a much more open and aware situation than I would have imagined possible.

HELEEN (HOLLAND)

I believe in everything that is good. I'm coming from a Roman Catholic family and I had to go to church when I was young. I never understood how people could be of different belief and all believe in God. I believe in God, but I don't believe in all those beliefs – all different and fighting – I just don't understand that.

I feel honoured when I hear the mother of my best friend, she says prayers for me. I think that's a beautiful thing. I even believe that I will start praying one day and I think that's good as well. I've got so many things to do and it's just there's no time for it.

Some find their religious beliefs strengthened.

ELIZABETH (UGANDA)

When I saw my husband deteriorating, the only thing to do was to surrender our lives to our Creator.

I had never seen somebody dying, so when he cried out in pain, I found myself helpless. The only help that was near me was the Holy Bible. I put it where he was showing me he had pain, asking God to relieve him of his pain. And God heard me cry, because as soon as I put it there, he immediately went to sleep. I thought he had gone to a normal sleep, not knowing that he had breathed his last. I am so grateful to that Creator that he took my husband in a peaceful way.

After I was diagnosed positive, I kept assuring my relations that I had been healed by a divine power. They saw my faith and they accepted the situation as it is. They know that, according to my faith, I shall live long with the virus. I believe that the Lord has the power to put it to an end, all one needs is strong belief in Him.

Generally I am enjoying a better life than what I enjoyed before. I was very happy with my husband, but this is a different Christian life I am living. I feel it's a much better life. It's consoling, it's nice to know that there is Someone who cares, Someone you can't see but He cares.

I believe whoever does something good for me, it is God who has gone through that person to assist me. And people have been assisting me. A lot of miracles have been happening in my life, unexpected. So many young people are finishing studying and they are still walking in the street, but my daughter got a job right away. Which I believe came from God as a provider.

It is a spirit right inside us, it's not the body that matters, the body can fade away, but when the spirit is strong you can live longer.

Some experience a kind of spiritual struggle.

KRISTINA (FINLAND)

I've been a Christian ten years. First, I prayed all the time – God heal me, God heal me, why don't you heal me? Every six months, I went to the doctor and they checked the blood. I was waiting that there is no HIV virus any more in my blood, but there is still.

But then I understand that He loves me the way I am. I'm HIV and He loves me. I read the Bible, that's the love of God.

I used to be very strict, but now I begin to understand more what is God's grace. That He really loves you, though you are what you are. We were told that God loves everybody, but it wasn't tested. But now I'm in this situation, I know that He loves me. That's a test, that's where you find out, you have to face your own fears and everything.

It was such a shock to me when I heard that I've got HIV, because Christians don't commit sin – I did, being with a man before marriage. In the Bible, it says that the wages of sin is death. It's true, of course, the wages of sin is death. But we cannot say that because I commit sin, that's why I've got HIV. People who have cancer, they have done wrong things, but they have done also good things. And it's not because of that they have got cancer.

It's a big monster, HIV. People can reject you, it's thought to be shameful. Many people are ashamed that they have HIV, they feel guilty. Sometimes I feel very guilty. I've been working on that, that I shouldn't feel guilty. It could happen to anybody. Small children get HIV and they are innocent.

ON DEATH AND DYING

It is often the first time that people think seriously about their own death.

REBECCA (ENGLAND)

Whenever I'd considered death before, I imagined that it was something that I would worry about in fifty years' time – not now. So the process I went through initially was coming to terms with my own mortality, with the fact that I had an illness that meant I was going to die. It was actually just accepting that I was mortal.

There was also a real sense of loss – grieving for lost time, the thought that I don't have a long future. You have to bring your life into the present tense. I can't say, 'When I'm thirty-five, I want to be doing this', because there's no guarantee of me being alive at thirty-five. I felt I'd lost my life.

Also, with HIV, the process of dying is a little frightening, because it's quite a slow painful death. You don't know what illness is going to get you. I have periods of trying to decide which one I would prefer. I would quite like to be aware of what's happening, so I can make decisions about it.

I think death will be easier for me than it will be for the people who love me, because they'll have to live with loss. A lot of my feelings about my death are focused around my partner being on his own after I'm gone. I worry a lot about him and I worry about my family.

KRISTINA (FINLAND)

The crisis when hearing that you have HIV is, some day you are going to die. Everybody's going to die, but somehow we know that it's over there. Nobody knows how long time we live, but it's different when you hear it.

You have to live with it. Sometimes, I feel like giving up, but I wouldn't kill myself. When you're very, very depressed, you feel like giving up. It's regressing – the feeling like a child that someone else must take care of me. But you have to grow up, be responsible, be adult.

HELEEN (HOLLAND)

I think I'm going to lose this battle. I want to be strong, but I think I'm going to die of it. I prefer to die in this way than running under a bus. Then, it's finished, boomp – you can't prepare anything, you can't think about it, you can't think about the past, what you want to do, nothing.

I think you must be realistic. I think when you're positive – and I'm very positive – that you will hold on very long. But I don't believe there is coming any medicine. I'm sorry, I don't think so. I think this must be one time we're losing the battle.

DANNY (NORTHERN IRELAND)

One of the people at college asked me, 'How long have you got?' Well, it was a question I'd asked myself at the early stages of my diagnosis. HIV equals AIDS equals death. There was a story I heard about a person living with AIDS for many years, coming out of the hospital after his regular check-up and the stupid so-and-so didn't look as he crossed the road and along came a bus and it killed him.

So nowadays if somebody asks me how long have I got – I don't want to be glib about it, because it's not a glib thing – but I ask, 'How long have *you* got?' Who's to know? I'm going to make jolly sure that I look right and left while I'm crossing the road, just in case there's something coming along that might kill me.

DAVID (ENGLAND)

I'm not afraid of dying any more. I've come to appreciate that death is something very natural. Pain's a much more difficult thing to endure. I get quite angry about death-denying. People don't like talking about death. We need to talk about it, I think.

My funeral's been planned about eight times, I keep changing my mind. My own dying is something I actually look forward to, because I've had a fab life.

Those with dependent children have particular anxieties.

ELIZABETH (UGANDA)

We were not rich, we were average people. Sometimes when my husband used to travel, he could buy the children nice clothes. We managed to get them to the best schools. Now when I thought of such children, who had been brought up in such a way, taking them to slums, it hurt me so much.

I'm involved in planning a house for my children. So that even if I pass away, they would have a house of their own to live in. That's taking all my energy and thoughts and feelings. I even go to the extent of not eating the way I should, because of sparing every penny to prepare the house.

I can't relax, I can't sleep well, all the time I imagine, 'Supposing it happened now, how would I leave my children?'

ANGELA (SCOTLAND)

The main issue was what was going to happen to my kids. That was what I used to really worry about. Just dying and the kids being left. I did have a friend that said she would take them and it made things a bit easier. But she has now got three kids of her own, so I think that's out of the window.

Now, my friend is trying to set up a group, like they've got in London, and we are trying to get rights for mums to plan things for their kids – now, before they take ill. Like foster mums, people they can have weekend relationships with every so often. And if anything did happen to the mum or dad, that's who they would end up with when the time came.

Some have already seen family and friends die.

ROSA (URUGUAY)

My story goes back to 1988, when my husband Miguel and I were told that we were both HIV-positive. He had already been suffering from health problems not related to the virus – an accident which fractured some vertebrae, chronic asthma and recurrent lung infections. He lost weight, was very depressed and his defences were diminishing. But it was not a very alarming picture. It was anyway a love story, where together we were both facing death from AIDS.

Then his doctors diagnosed AIDS and they were pessimistic about his future. The information we had was that AIDS was an inexorably fatal disease and that patients would last only a very short period. The doctors we consulted corroborated this and gave us no hope for Miguel. He was advised to confront death in the near future.

Miguel died in the emergency department of a Buenos Aires hospital in September 1988. When we arrived at the hospital, I told the staff that he needed an urgent operation, because he had an intestinal obstruction. The surgeon decided to do nothing, arguing that he did not have the necessary type of blood and that the operation was highly risky anyway. I urged him to go ahead and operate and that I was assuming total responsibility. The surgeon gave me no answer and left.

A while later I found him talking nervously with another doctor. I asked him again to save my husband's life. Both doctors looked down silently and told me to wait. It was late at night. They left us alone and nobody dared to come near us. Time was running out and Miguel was getting worse. I recalled the doctor and he sent me out of the room, saying they were going to apply some heart massage. I rejected the idea of leaving my husband alone, as we had been together throughout his illness. The doctors insisted again that I should leave the room. As I gave them an emphatic no, they called the police. These doctors who had refused to save a life in the face of a hypothetical risk to themselves were now fearing that I would attack them! Finally, Miguel died while I was holding his hand and, ironically, instead of being surrounded by doctors, we were watched by a policeman.

JOSEPH (UGANDA)

In June 1987, I had never heard about AIDS. I was a post-graduate student at the University of Nairobi, happily married with two children, aged four and six months.

In October, something unusual happened – an attack of herpes zoster on my wife. She was taken to hospital, treated and discharged after two weeks. We continued as normal for some time. When I finished the course, I went back to Uganda. In July 1988, my wife was down with recurrent fever. In December, she was down with high fever. In January, her relatives opted to steal her away so she could be treated by a witch doctor. There was demand for white goats, very lean, and several thousand shillings for a cure. I sold a car and other properties, but there was nothing good done to her health.

After some time, I met a friend, now dead, who advised me to take an HIV test. The following day I took a test. The results, of course, were positive. I hurried home to inform my wife and the following day we went together to get her test. Indeed, it was positive. On 1st November, she passed away.

GRACE (ZIMBABWE)

I fell pregnant in February 1988. A friend advised me to abort, because she feared for my health. I had lost weight and was feeling very weak, but decided against an abortion.

The birth was complicated and painful. The nurses feared they were going to lose both mother and child. However, a girl was born, but showed signs of failure to grow. The baby showed signs of infection, had diarrhoea and pneumonia on and off. Treatments did not seem to help.

It was not easy to care for the baby. I knew my daughter would not live, and after seven months, she passed away. This was painful, but inevitable. I get reminded if I see some children of my daughter's age.

DAVID (ENGLAND)

I've buried twenty-six of my friends since January this year. I just wonder how any of us are dealing with the loss and the horror of that.

I'd never had a garden until three years ago. It's become the obsession of my life, where I can work out what it's all about. I can find answers in the garden that bring me peace. When I have those dark moments, when my friends die, I think there is my garden – the roses and all sorts of things planted in memory of them – and that's great.

There is little expectation of an early cure.

REBECCA (ENGLAND)

Sometimes I have a fantasy about it. I know a lot of other women who are HIV-positive and I have a fantasy of us all being together and getting the news that we have some cure, some way out of this nightmare. It would all be over. But I can't get rid of HIV, it's not going to go away. I don't feel that there will be a miraculous cure within the next five years.

The AZT is prolonging my period of health. I have this image that when AZT isn't helping any more, then I'll have ddI. Hopefully, I'll be able to hang on long enough, buying time for the next drug, the next thing. They are much better at treating the problems you get, but there's nothing really concrete to believe in at the moment.

I get very frustrated about the situation with drugs. It seems a very slow process. The combination treatments with AZT and ddC look very promising. But the chances of us getting treated with those drugs in the next two years are virtually nil, because of the long testing procedures. Long-term side effects are not really an issue for me. If I get cancer in ten years because I've been taking AZT, I would be grateful to have lived that long.

ERIK (SWEDEN)

They'll find a cure, but now not, not in five years' time. Maybe ten years' time, fifteen years' time. This is a very difficult nut to crack. We have seen how long it has taken with cancer. I know it's all speeded up a bit, but I think that's a realistic time to expect something.

We could be lucky. At times, I think I might live to see a cure, the little pill that can stop my infection. But I don't really believe that I will live to see that day. I must prepare for living the rest of my life as an HIV-positive.

THE FUTURE

Having HIV does not mean that there is no future.

IMRAT (MALAYSIA)

Number one, I don't intend to die yet. I still want to live. I have plans. I want to work, to buy a house for myself. I just started a job a month ago, a permanent job. I need a steady income – I never felt better and I don't see any reason why I should not have a permanent job. It's full-time and I am looking for promotion in that job.

I'm healthy, there's nothing wrong with me. Some people will say, 'You have HIV, you're sick', but I don't think that way. To me, HIV is just like 'flu – it'll go away some day, if you don't think about it.

KRISTINA (FINLAND)

I decided that now it's a good time to go to study. I couldn't continue any more where I was working. It would have been too much for me. But now at school I can be quite myself. It's been very good, very interesting. I enjoy my study very much. I don't think so much about HIV.

I want to express myself more. I'd like to start dancing and express myself in that way. And to draw, to write poems. School is a very good place for that. We had to write a short story for children and a poem. I wrote a story about burial from a child's point of view – how a small child would react, watching all those things going on, Grandmama has now died. That was one way I was expressing myself and my feelings.

When I finish my studies, I have an idea that I work with AIDS or HIV children, but there are not many in Finland, maybe two or three. I don't know. I am afraid that if I go to ordinary kindergarten, I can't do that work – if people know that I'm HIV, they could fire me.

I see optimism that I can cope, although I have HIV. I can still manage, I can take care of myself. I love myself more than before, I can accept myself, I grow as a person.

DAVID (ENGLAND)

I feel as if my life's much more spacious than it's ever been before. I've got much more time. And I find it much easier to pray, much easier to open myself up to things beyond the immediate. So there's a spaciousness in my life which feels like a rootedness that's important.

I remember for weeks I was just preparing to die. And then you suddenly realize you're not going to die. What do you do? What do you plan for – how long ahead? Well now, of course, my partner and I plan for ever – well, he was given two years to live four and a half years ago. There's a sense in which we've brought into our lives living for ever and dying now and saying, well, that's how it is.

And somehow one step at a time. But let's have a future and let's have some vision of hope. Not being a victim, but moving into being some kind of person whose life is powerful because I am taking charge of it. Not handing over to the doctors, not handing over to the Church, not handing over to anybody else what I can do for myself.

HELEEN (HOLLAND)

Everybody needs help, everybody finds it in his way. I went back to Holland and found other people and an organization. I talk with people coming in first time and I am sitting on a telephone helpline. And helping with organizing events. I like it very much, I like meeting other people.

But I'm getting very tired of it. I've had enough of HIV. I had an overdose of HIV for the last year or so and I want to change it now.

I believe in myself, I think I should stop drinking, stop smoking, go and meditate. I should go and do more work on myself. I have been too busy with HIV and other people. It's easy for me to do something for other people, rather than for myself. I must push to go back and work on myself.

MARTIN (AUSTRALIA)

You feel that you want to contribute something, to make a difference. After three years, I feel that I'm stagnating on a personal level. I now need to move away from it, if I'm going to deal with some of the issues that I'm identifying now.

It started to occur to me that I might have to deal with a period of being sick. It's not death, it's *dying* that concerns me. Because dying involves disability and dependency. I've got to resolve all these things. Or get to a point where I feel I'm able to deal with it. I think that it's time that I became realistic about what might happen.

The work I'm doing, it's just AIDS all the time. I feel tired by AIDS, the whole issue. It can drain you. The support you get from your colleagues is very seductive, especially if you're HIV-positive. The issue sucks you in. It was the best thing I could have done at the time. But it takes it out of you. I need to get away from it, to do other things.

I need to just stop and sit quietly for quite a long time and figure out what has happened to me over the last four years. I don't think I've given myself a chance to do that. Everything has been so frantic. I need to stop.

I've been so wrapped up in the job and the politics and my

relationship. And on a personal level, I guess I am frightened. Something is going to change in my life and my approach to my life. I feel it coming.

ADVICE TO OTHERS

Everyone has to find the path which is best for him- or herself. But here are a few words of advice to those who have just discovered that they have HIV.

WINSTON (CANADA)

My advice is, take your time. Everything you feel is honest. It's not a death sentence, don't think it's the end. Most people who become HIV-positive stop living. They become obsessed with it and forget about doing the things that they enjoy in their life.

You must maintain living. Dying is too damn easy, it's *living* that's hard. That's the reality and that's my advice – to recognize what you're feeling and go with it.

MARY (ZIMBABWE)

I should be welcoming them and then show them that I am very happy about them, about what they are. First of all, I *don't* tell them you are going to develop AIDS or you are going to die. There are some people who are HIV-positive, but they don't develop AIDS, they continue living.

REBECCA (ENGLAND)

What I found to be the most helpful when I was first diagnosed was to meet other people who are HIV. That is consoling. You mostly meet people who look really well, so that can take away a lot of the fear. But also you don't feel you're the only person that this has happened to.

And it's sensible to get informed medically. It can be very frightening, but it is sensible. I have met people who are so frightened that they don't go to hospital appointments, they don't read anything to do with HIV and AIDS. But although sometimes you read about terrible illnesses you might get, it is actually very sensible.

There are things you can do to protect yourself and there are treatments that are effective – not necessarily that deal with the virus – but treatments that are very effective for skin conditions, for pneumonia. It's only since I found out I had HIV that I've got the right treatment for my skin, having lived with this eczema on my face all the time.

KRISTINA (FINLAND)

Nobody should give up, if he hears that he has HIV. He should not give up, but start taking care of himself and face his fears. And not run away.

It's important that one makes clear his attitude towards death. Because death is hidden in Western countries. When people are dying, they are taken to hospitals, they don't die at home any more. Children haven't seen a dead person. You have to make clear, what is your attitude.

MONIKA (GERMANY)

I feel everybody has to go his own way. I would say to them, find out your own way. Find out what you want and *do* it. I didn't feel I was doing what I wanted to do. So I would give them the advice to look what they want to do and to do it.

And neglect good advices from the outside.

DAVID (ENGLAND)

I don't know if I'd give advice. I try not to give advice, because I think everyone's got to make their own journey.

There might come a time when I could introduce the idea that you don't have to die as a result of being diagnosed HIV-positive. And maybe even it's a gift that can enable you to make your life what you'd always hoped it might be.

I wouldn't give that as advice to a newly diagnosed person. I'd just give them my love and hope that would open a way for them.

IF YOU WANT TO LOVE ME

If you want to love me
Then love me now.
Don't look for tomorrow
And don't ask me how.
I can't give you a guideline—
It is your love,
Your life,
It is you.

If you want to leave me,
Then leave me now.
Don't think about me
And don't ask how.
I can't give you peace
You don't have inside.
It is your peace,
Your life,
It is you.

If you want to paint me
In your dreams,
Don't start thinking
With 'it seems'.
It is your dream,
Your life,
It is you.

And if you want to try to be
Just a little bit like me
And ask me how—
Just start now
To live your life,
Find your peace,
Love your love
And be you.

Dietmar Bolle, 1990

PEOPLE IN THIS BOOK

Interviewed	AGE	DATE OF DIAGNOSIS
Europe		
Angela (Scotland)	34	1986
Ben (England)	46	1984
Danny (Northern Ireland)	32	1990
David (England)	44	1985
Erik (Sweden)	27	1983
Heleen (Holland)	34	1989
Kristina (Finland)	28	1990
Lucia (Italy)	25	1984
Monika (Germany)	25	1985
Pavel (Czechoslovakia)	44	1987
Rebecca (England)	26	1990
Sarah (mother of Daisy) (England)	37	1985
USA and Canada		
Mark (Canada)	25	1987
Peter (USA)	53	1986
Winston (Canada)	31	1982
Latin America		
Roberto (Mexico)	43	1986
Asia and Australia		
Dominic (India)	32	1989
Imrat (Malaysia)	28	1985
Martin (Australia)	31	1987

Africa

Elizabeth (Uganda)	48	1990
Mary (Zimbabwe)	25	1987

Others Quoted

Europe
Boris (Bulgaria)
Derek (England)
Josie (England)
Philip (England)
Pierre (Belgium)
Umberto (Italy)

USA and Canada
Paul (USA)

Latin America
Fernando (Brazil)
Juan (Colombia)
Rosa (Uruguay)

Africa
Alice (Botswana)
Angelina (Uganda)
Benjamin (Uganda)
Grace (Zimbabwe)
Jennifer (Uganda)
Jonathan (Uganda)
Joseph (Uganda)
Joshua (Zambia)
Martha (Uganda)
Michael (South Africa)
Prudence (Botswana)
Rashid (Morocco)
Stephen (Uganda)